SURVIVE THE 20TH CENTURY DIET

SCIENTIFIC SOLUTIONS TO A DIET GONE WRONG

A "New" Abridged Edition of
GREEN LEAVES OF BARLEY; NATURE'S MIRACLE REJUVENATOR

by Dr. Mary Ruth Swope

WITH DAVID A. DARBRO, M.D.

SURVIVING THE 20TH CENTURY DIET
A 'New' Abridged Edition of;
Green Leaves of Barley: Nature's Miracle Rejuvenator

Copyright © 1996 by Dr. Mary Ruth Swope
Swope Enterprises
P.O. Box 62104, Phoenix, AZ 85082-2104

ISBN 09606936-6-1

Library of Congress Cataloging in Publication Data

Cover design by Tom Paliga
Typography by Gray Matters Design, Mesa, Arizona
Printed in the United States of America

Published and distributed by
Swope Enterprises
P.O. Box 62104, Phoenix, AZ 85082-2104
1-800-447-9772 or (602) 275-7957

Acknowledgments

The major responsibility for creating this abridged version of the book, *Green Leaves of Barley Nature's Miracle Rejuvenator,* was done by my skilled editor, Val Cindric of Delmont, PA. Without her consistently challenging and fruitful suggestions, I would not have completed this work in 1996.

I am grateful to a number of friends who contributed to the writing of the original Green Leaves of Barley book, published first in 1987. Their names are listed in the acknowledgments page of that work.

I am especially indebted to my faithful friend and secretary, Charlotte Bates, for her dedicated work. And to my step-granddaughter, Elise Darbro, I am deeply grateful for her proofreading and editing of the book in its final stages.

As always, I am deeply grateful to God for strength, health, life and my years of education and professional experiences, all needed for a work of this magnitude.

Other books by Dr. Mary Ruth Swope:

• *Are You Sick & Tired of Feeling Sick & Tired?*
• *Listening Prayer*
• *Green Leaves of Barley. A Food With Real Power*
• *Spiritual Roots of Barley*
• *Bless Your Children Every Day*
• *Some Gold Nuggets in Nutrition*

Contents

Introduction

Millions of Americans are waking up to the fact that they are in less than excellent health. In addition to realizing that they do not understand how it happened, they are becoming keenly aware of the limited knowledge available of how to correct their acquired poor health.

Many people are disenchanted with the medical profession's persistent use of pharmaceuticals without the possibility of a choice of treatment modalities. We hope to offer light (without "heat") that will benefit multitudes of people.

You may be asking: "What happened to my health?"—and "What can I do about it?" This book will attempt to answer these two questions with special emphasis on the green leaves of barley as an ideal food concentrate for helping to correct the problem.

You will find a vast array of subjects, related to powdered barley leaves, thoroughly covered in an easy-to-understand manner from reliable sources of information, including recent research studies. My daughter, Susan Darbro, helps lay the groundwork for understanding why our bodies need the nutrients in this miracle rejuvenator.

If you follow the advice given here, you can really "feel the difference" in your health.

Dr. David A. Darbro, my son-in-law, will get you headed in the right direction as he relates his own struggle in the battle between orthodox medicine and alternative medicine.

There is no attempt in this book to answer every conceivable question about the 20th Century diet of North Americans. The goal is to present some of the major inadequacies of our diet and to offer what the author feels has been scientifically proven as the best antidote for poor nutrition — i.e., organically grown (without artificial fertilizers and pesticides), unprocessed, fresh, raw foods and food concentrates, especially the green leaves of barley as offered by Dr. Yoshihide Hagiwara.

CHAPTER I

The Physician *"Within"* Knows Best

By David A. Darbro, M.D.

After I graduated from medical school, I spent 15 years doing just what I had been taught: to prescribe drugs, and say, "I'll see you in two weeks." Gradually, I began to realize my patients never actually got well. If they had high blood pressure, for instance, I could control it by giving them appropriate medication, but the problem itself would return the minute the medication was discontinued.

One day, it dawned on me that all I had accomplished in spending five years and thousands of dollars in medical schools was that I had learned how to maintain disease at an acceptable level. The problem is not how the medical system operates in its own context— which in America is the best in the world — but how it fails to maintain health.

COMMON SENSE MEDICINE

The earliest medicine was practiced from an empirical standpoint — you might call it the common-sense method. I see something that works, so I do it. I might not understand why it works, but the fact that it does work is more important to me than the explanation why.

Hippocrates, called the Father of Medicine, believed the body was capable of healing itself. As a result, his goal was to promote the general wellness of the body so that it would be strong enough to rid itself of a particular disease. In this tradition of medicine, the overall state of health is addressed, and the goal becomes the strengthening of our adaptive powers - the common sense way! This was known as Empiricism.

Ancient Greece produced another viewpoint from which has arisen the medical giants of today. Eventually, this way of thought came into conflict with the healing arts previously mentioned. By the early nineteenth century, the two traditions were locked in combat.

The empiricists practiced a form of medicine called homeopathy. We do not, even today, understand the mechanism behind the success of this treatment, but it is an undeniable fact it worked — and still does. Although homeopathy didn't conform to the rational traditions of medicine, it got results.

What is the essential difference between these two approaches to medicine? Empiricists use "similars," and rationalists use "opposites."

The health practitioner who uses similars wants to gently stimulate the patient's healing responses, or physis. He doesn't want to upset the "balance" any more than it is already upset.

The rationalist tradition, however, doesn't think in terms of promoting health but rather in terms of fighting disease.

For example, if a person with a diarrhea problem comes to a physician's office and says, "Doc, I've got the runs. What should I do?"

If his doctor is from the rationalist's school (which 99.9 percent of American doctors are), he will very likely prescribe a drug that slows up the movement of the bowel. Since diarrhea is caused by too much bowel activity, he will treat it with the opposite—a substance to slow its normal activity down to almost nothing.

If, however, the patient's doctor is from the empirical approach, he might suggest a very gentle enema to cleanse out the bowel — an action similar to how the body is already coping with this particular imbalance.

NO COMPETITION ALLOWED

The history of medical practice in our country took a very sad turn in 1849, the year the American Medical Association was founded. Homeopathic physicians, who were considered the "enemy," were barred from membership in the AMA. As a result, within 60 years there was a "near-total uniformity to American medicine, with hardly a dissenting voice to be heard."[1]

With the coming of the Civil War, another major change in the face of medicine took place — the rise of the pharmaceutical industry.

Prior to this time, doctors themselves were familiar with and mixed the ingredients they prescribed for their patients. Now the compounding of medicines became centralized, and doctors no longer needed to bother learning their own business. Pharmaceutic companies not only identified their products but also indicated to the physician which disease was to be "cured" by which particular product. Within a very few years, there were literally thousands of patented medicines.

As a result, some pharmaceutical houses supplied pharmacists with the financing, pamphlets, and supplies to begin their businesses. With the drug industry supporting both pharmacists and physicians, it had no competition. Medicine gradually evolved into a "drug-industry-oriented treatment philosophy."[2]

I am the first to admit that pharmaceuticals have saved thousands of lives and certainly have a valid place in the practice of medicine. In fact, I prescribe them myself. But when we look at drugs in the larger context of the healing arts, we come up with some major problems.

THE BOOK OF SIDE EFFECTS

Even the pharmaceutical industry itself recognizes the obvious: For each desired action of a drug, there are usually numerous undesired actions — "side effects." Published annually, the *Physicians' Desk Reference* catalogues all the drugs on the market, giving information on how they work, when they should be used, when they should not be used, and warnings and adverse reactions based upon testing with real people.

I am not opposed to using prescription drugs when the need arises, but my point here is that they are dangerous substances and should be used later rather than sooner.

Because the toxicity of drugs is so well known, one of the major tasks of a physician's work is to assess what we call the "risk-benefit factor." In other words, we need to figure out if we harm the patient more by giving the drug or by withholding it. Most weapons against disease are also weapons against health.

Sadly, there is much truth to the statement, "We cured the disease, but lost the patient." This is a tragic commentary on a profession dedicated to the saving of human life.

DIET AND DISEASE

As a physician, I realized I was maintaining acceptable disease rather than promoting health. It's essential to grasp that distinction. Anti-disease is *not* the same as pro-health.

The more I studied, the more I began to see that my methods had to change. I had to do much less of fighting disease and do much more of promoting wellness — so my patients, true to Hippocrates' wisdom, can heal themselves.

Modern medicine is responsible for eradicating a host of diseases in which micro-organisms are the primary cause. Polio, smallpox, tuberculosis, and cholera, for example, are rarely if ever seen today. Yet, we still have disease.

If medicine has done such a good job of stamping out disease, why are health care costs in the billions of dollars every year? And why are physicians ignoring the use of nutrition as a treatment modality when it is a well-known fact that "70 percent of all deaths in the United States are caused by diseases linked to the consumption of our diet"?[3]

THE BIGGEST KILLERS

Medicine has done a wonderful job of stamping out a certain kind of disease — the acute kind. But what kills us these days are chronic degenerative diseases. What does that mean? It means that the "Big Four" killers — heart disease, cancer, diabetes, and atherosclerosis — develop gradually over a period of years.

The problem isn't that a patient is at the wrong place at the wrong time and catches a "fatal bug." **The problem is that an unhealthy lifestyle and an unhealthy environment slowly but steadily erode the general state of wellness, causing the body to slowly deteriorate until one day the danger signals can no longer be ignored.**

It might seem as if the patient suddenly dropped dead of a heretofore nonexistent heart problem, but that's not what really happened. The patient had a high fat, high sugar diet for years, and it was slowly but surely clogging up his arteries. He smoked cigarettes, which caused the vessels to become even smaller. He was under stress for 20 years with a job he didn't like, causing his body to work much harder than it should have. His primary form of exercise was leaving his easy chair to go raid the refrigerator during commercial breaks on TV. He suddenly dropped dead, even though he'd just been to his doctor and checked out fine!

Chronic degenerative disease needs to be reversed — not by drugs and surgeries, but by the changing of lifestyles and environments — by promoting what is healthy. What does this best — traditional doctoring or alternative medicine?

PROOF OR REALITY?

Much of what I've learned since my "awakening" has to do with using nutrition as medicine. Because many alternative therapies require patient awareness and lifestyle changes, they cannot always be "proven" as defined by the scientific community. As one famous physician astutely put it, "It is easier to cure a hundred incurables than it is to prove that the treatment works."[4]

Anyone who wants to have vibrant health and be "disease free" must study and apply the scientifically-proven principles of nutrition. There is absolutely no other way to achieve a constant state of wellness. **All living, rejuvenating, healing processes are intimately related to the work of nutrients.**

The whole world has served as a proving ground for this concept. What humans (or animals for that matter) regularly consume in terms of their food and drink can be used as a remarkably accurate predictor of their length and quality of life, their reproductibility, their size, vitality, disease patterns, mental problems, productivity, and so forth.

America is no exception to this. Our diet for the past 50 years has provided convincing evidence, if not conclusive proof, that by accepting a poorer quality diet than our ancestors, we have lowered our standards of health.

One doctor is quoted as saying, "If we eat wrongly, no doctor can cure us — if we eat rightly, no doctor is needed."

Hippocrates, the "father of medicine" is credited as saying, **"Food is your best medicine and the best foods are the best medicines."** The natural forces within us are truly the healers of disease.

In the chapters that follow, you will discover a remarkable "nutrient booster" that will help you help your body survive the American diet.

CHAPTER II

Wake up, America ...
You're Sick!

We have a choice to make when we shop for medical care. Are we going to accept the "mostly drugstore" or the "mostly drugless" variety of treatment?

I suggest we shop at the "nutrient pharmacy" for as much of our cell/tissue/organ needs as is possible — and accept drugs only in case of acute illness. As one doctor is quoted as saying, **"If we eat wrongly, no doctor can cure us - if we eat rightly, no doctor is needed." Make "wellness" instead of "controlled illness" your lifetime goal.**

In a recent seminar on orthomolecular medicine — which means the use of nutrition in the treatment of illnesses — my eyes were opened to the truth about the health of Americans in a new way: Americans are epidemically sick and need to wake up and wise up to the reasons for their unhealthiness.

Included here are a few of the facts pinpointed at the conference.

WHY ARE AMERICANS DYING?

Americans are spending around $210 billion annually on heart disease, $14 billion on cancer, $10 billion on diabetes and, now, $8 billion in Medicare alone on osteoporosis (porous bones).

1. Heart Disease. According to the *Statistical Abstracts of the United States, 1992* nearly one million Americans die annually from heart disease. This might not appear shocking, unless we know how these figures compare with those at the turn of this century. There were very few deaths from heart disease then. In fact, the first article to appear in the *Journal of the American Medical Association* on this subject was in 1911.

Why, in less than 85 years, have we gone from just a few people dying annually from heart disease, to nearly one million? The answer is not simple, but it definitely involves changes in our eating habits.

2. Cancer. Deaths from cancer have also been climbing steadily since the turn of this century. In 1992 more than one-half million people died from cancer. That figure was up 225 percent since 1960! Why? The American Institute of Cancer Research estimated in 1984 that as many as 60 percent of these cases could be related to *diet!*

3. Diabetes Mellitus While diabetes has been identified as a sickness since the time of the Greeks, it is only since the turn of this century that it has become rampant. About 10 million Americans now have active cases, with nearly 600,000 new cases reported annually. Again, this illness is related to our diet.

Two physicians studying diabetes have made similar public statements about this disease. They said, in essence, that if patients were to lower their weight to normal and keep it there, adult-onset diabetes would disappear in slightly more than 80 percent of the cases. Losing extra pounds will also lower high blood pressure in the majority of cases and improve stamina and resistance to many other diseases.

4. Osteoporosis. This is a condition once only identified with grandmothers. These elderly women, far past menopause, often suffered broken hips because the hip socket became so spongy it wouldn't hold the body's weight. Their hips break and then they fall, in 80 percent or more of the cases.

The United States now holds the world record for osteoporosis. Approximately 30 percent of women past menopause have it, and, for the first time in our history, it is also being found in young women and in men.

These facts are unheard of in many countries. Why? What is happening in America that isn't happening in other countries?

TWO CULPRITS: MEAT AND SOFT DRINKS

Many research studies allude to the fact that high phosphorus and/or phosphoric acid (found in meat and soft drinks) pulls calcium out of the bony structures (bones, teeth, and nails) in the process of digestion and assimilation. This has a disastrous effect on bone density, leaving them porous and spongy.

According to the National Soft Drink Association, in 1993 soft drink consumption has increased to the point that Americans are consuming 51.8 gallons per person per year. That compares to 10.4 in 1950.

At the same time, consumption of meat, poultry, and fish hit an all-time high in 1993. According to USDA figures, per capita consumption reached 221.7 pounds — a figure 19 percent above the previous 75-year average of 186 pounds.[1]

I believe these two changes in the American diet are largely responsible for our extremely high incidence of osteoporosis.

DEGENERATIVE DISEASES: REALLY BIG BUSINESS!

Degenerative diseases are epidemic in America. In fact, you or someone you know probably suffers from one or more of these health problems:

• **Kidney Stones.** The incidence of kidney stones in the U.S. has doubled in the past 20 years. The cause, in 75 percent of these cases, is thought to be related to our high sucrose (white sugar) consumption.

Two to five hours after heavy sugar intake, there is a burst of two times the amount of calcium released into the urine. Another cause is our high acid-ash diet due to high meat intake. When calcium is pulled from the bones, it is released through the kidneys, resulting in stone formation before it is excreted.

• *Gallstones.* About 1,000 Americans are operated on daily for this condition. In Africa, according to Dr. Dennis Burkett, there have been two cases in the past 20 years!

• *Dental Cavities.* Almost every American has them; we consider deteriorating teeth "normal." In many parts of the world, you couldn't find a single case to show a dentist.

• *Prostate Gland Problems.* About 70 percent of American men over 60 years of age have this problem. We hold the international record in this category!

• *Ulcerative Colitis.* Two million of us have it. It is unknown in many parts of the world.

• *Gastrointestinal Problems.* Billions of dollars are spent on over-the-counter products and prescribed drugs for our belching, bloating, flatulence, and constipation.

• *Vericose Veins And Hemorrhoids.* These problems are now epidemic among us. More fiber and exercise would help prevent and/or alleviate these cases.

• *Hypertension.* Thirty million Americans have it and are being medicated with drugs costing billions of dollars. Just 30 years ago it was an uncommon problem.

• *Gout and Arthritis.* Millions in our society are now receiving medication to alleviate suffering from these two conditions. Traditionally diseases of the elderly, these conditions now encompass all age groups, including young children. Recent figures show one in seven to have some form of arthritis, costing us $13 billion annually in medical care and lost wages.[2]

• *Diverticulitis.* This is another disease with strong dietary implications, and it is epidemic in the United States. However, in countries where fiber has not been removed from food supplies, it is practically unheard of.

• *Iatrogenic Diseases* (M.D. Induced). These are some of the saddest cases to me. All drugs have side-effects, and there is no known antidote for effecting a cure in many cases. Millions are ill because of this.

• *Hyperactivity.* This condition affects millions in our society and is a condition which has not come of age yet! No cases were known as little as 20 years ago!

• *Allergies.* These are big business for our medical doctors. Millions are ill from these hard-to-diagnose and harder still to cure allergies to foods, drugs, and chemicals.

• *Atherosclerosis And Arteriosclerosis.* These conditions are household words today. Millions of Americans have faulty circulation and hardening of the arteries.

• *Cirrhosis of the Liver.* This is as much an epidemic in America as one of its major causes — heavy drinking of alcoholic beverages. About 6 percent of our population is now classified as "escape drinkers." Teenage alcoholism is greatly increasing. Some physicians today say the rising rate of liver damage among even the very young can be traced to the appalling consumption of soft drinks. It is safe to say that the need to maintain the health of one's liver ranks at the top of the list.

• *Mental Illness.* This condition is also increasing among us. About half of our diseases are thought to originate from our minds and negative emotions — anxiety, fear, hate, jealousy, bitterness, unforgiveness, grief, and the like.

• *Hypoglycemia* and *Candida Albicans.* Physicians differ in opinion on these disorders. In fact, some still doubt the significance and/or prevalence of either condition. Most who treat them, however, would acknowledge that our high intake of sugar and refined carbohydrates is one of the basic offenders in both disorders.

SICKNESS IN THE MAKING

The diseases Americans suffer do not happen overnight. It takes years for the body to break down and permit disease to overtake us. Cancer can take as long as 20 years to develop. Heart disease can be 30 to 40 years in the making. Arthritis, kidney stones, osteoporosis, diabetes, hardening of the arteries, and many others fall into this category.

During the interim years, many people are not sick enough to be symptomatic. The symptoms are tiredness, depression, muscle pains, insomnia, lassitude, lack of motivation, and many other diffuse symptoms such as constipation, indigestion, gas, and headaches.

The symptoms that cause you to stop work and lie down in the sick bed, come later.

We are told that more than 100 million Americans are suffering from these "new degenerative diseases" to one degree or another. How can this be true?

We have more physicians of all types, more hospitals and clinics of various kinds, more highly specialized nursing services, more health spas, and more health-education programs than any country in the world. When compared to other nations, why are we not near the top now in terms of overall health?

The answer is not simple. Keep in mind that Americans live in the highly stressful fast lane on a seven-day-a-week basis. This is accompanied by a high intake of drugs (prescribed, over-the-counter, and on-the-street types) and by much smoking, alcohol abuse, and high levels of junk food intake. The modern-day air, water, and soil pollution also create tremendous assaults on our health, as do the negative lifestyle factors that cause the breakdown of DNA, RNA, and our immune systems. All of these play a part in our unwellness.

PREVENTION OR CURE?

One way to conserve or restore health is the use of natural remedies for fighting disease. Such things as charcoal, herbs, teas, hydrotherapy, heat and cold, fasting, massage, exercise, nutrients, foods, rest, and pure water are almost unheard of as treatment modalities.

Sadly for us, the standard medical procedure in America now includes only four approved treatment methods: prescription drugs, radiation, chemotherapy, and surgery. Legitimate research, as well as clinical observation and testimony, show these four treatment modalities should be used mostly for "crisis" medical treatment or as a last resort. They have very little effect in stopping the course of — much less preventing — our modern-day diseases.

Books like Dr. Robert Mendolsohn's *Confessions of a Medical Heretic and Medical Mayhem,* reveal that many highly trained physicians believe the drugs presently being used are poisonous and useless, if not lethal, to sick people. It is a well-documented fact that prescription drugs, even antibiotics, can be hazardous to your health.

DRUGS OR NUTRITION?

A 26-year-old friend of mine was diagnosed as being "hyper" and "nervous." Her physician prescribed the following drugs for these problems — Navane, Symmetrel, and Amitriptilyne.

What are the possible side effects of these drugs? Let me share a few: Rapid heartbeat, lightheadedness, low blood pressure, drowsiness, restlessness, insomnia, rash, itching, hives, exaggerated sunburn, dry mouth, blurred vision, nasal congestion, constipation, increased sweating, increased salivation, changes in appetite, nausea, vomiting, weakness, fatigue. Long-term use may lead to involuntary movements of the tongue, jaw, mouth, or face.

Does this stimulate you to learn about the possible side effects of the drugs *you* are taking? Maybe it will also encourage you to seek alternate treatment modalities for your symptoms.

Nutrition would be a first place for you to look. At least one thing is certain — proper nutrition has not one possibility of an iatrogenic (doctor induced) consequence. Foods in their natural state do not have damaging or life-threatening side effects. The side effect of totally natural foods, for example — fabulous health!

WHAT MAKES CANCER CELLS SPREAD?

The uselessness of surgery for cancer has been known for at least three decades. Your surgeon, of course, will be the last to admit it. But, it is well known in medical circles that surgery causes cancer cells to spread.

Doctors at Kaiser Hospital in California have shown radiation to cause new cancers to form where the X-rays of the first radiation burn normal tissue. After suffering the extreme nausea, weakness, hair loss, and general debilitation resulting from this radical treatment method, they are often worse than before the treatment.

What about chemotherapy? Studies have clearly shown this treatment has limited success in prolonging life for patients who undergo it. While it destroys cancer cells in the blood, it also damages healthy cells and generally weakens the immune system. In addition, chemotherapy causes cancer cells to grow stronger to fight the drug "offender."[3]

If Americans want to get well from cancer, heart disease, arthritis, diabetes, obesity, and a whole host of debilitating conditions, in my opinion, they will have to find non-orthodox treatment modalities involving nutrition and other remedies "provided by nature" as the major components.

The general public, to a growing extent, is now beginning to connect disease with dietary deficiencies or overindulgences. The medical profession, however, continues to ignore this association and neglects to seek answers where they can so easily be found — in foods and nutrition.

This is nothing new. Jesus told about a woman sick for 12 years with a hemorrhage. She had suffered from doctors, had become poor from paying them, and was no better, but, in fact, worse. (Matt. 9: 20-22)

NO MEDICAL CURE?

Americans are being denied freedom of choice in treatment modalities for our diseases. Doctors who disagree with standard medical procedure are being put in prison and denied the right to practice medicine if they ignore the rules of the "undercover dictatorship." Any kind of monopoly encourages poorer service at higher prices.

Perhaps this will change when the grass roots public refuses to accept the presently accepted standard medical procedures and opts for self-treatment or chooses to attend clinics outside of the continental United States, such as those in Mexico or Bermuda.

Each of us must take our own part in prevention much more seriously. Is it "merely a coincidence" that the conditions that have no medical cure are the ones we can and must take personal responsibility for preventing? The tragedy of degenerative disease is that the conditions which are so often fatal by the time they require attention from a doctor are the very same conditions that are almost entirely preventable through a personal commitment to good nutrition.

YOUR BEST WEAPON AGAINST DISEASE

We have almost buried our strongest and best weapon to fight disease, general malaise, and poor health — a fresh, healthy food supply grown on an organically fertilized soil without the aid of sophisticated chemicals. Our high-tech foods cannot be nutritionally compared to the foods we were growing and consuming in this nation at the turn of the century.

Today, a large part of what we eat can rightfully be called "foodless." Produced totally in manufacturers' laboratories, our foods are drugged, embalmed, dead, coal-tarred, artificial, skeletonized, polished, processed, refined, sterilized, oiled, sprayed, waxed, degenerated, unclean, frozen, canned, dried, impure junk — and now the threat of irradiated food.

All processed foods can be put down the esophagus with varying degrees of ease and pleasure, but they do not feed the cells with the nutrients required to create and sustain healthful bodies. Those come only from a "natural" food supply. An example is spray-dried green leaves of barley, which are organically grown without chemical fertilizers or pesticides and are not refined or processed with high heat or freezing.

Preventive-health-minded professionals urge us to eat whole-grain "natural" cereals in preference to those that have been highly altered by processing. Whole grains are natural, and anything natural is of better quality than that same food refined or processed.

SUGAR AND CAFFEINE

It has been estimated that in America today 65 percent of our foods are processed and 60 percent of us are epidemically sick! Is this one reason why?

Our most startling changes in food consumption have taken place since the 1950's. We are drinking more alcohol, beer, and soft drinks, but less water. The replacement of soft drinks for water to satisfy "anytime" and "all-the-time" thirst is the most tragic in terms of health.

Cola drinks are consumed daily in larger amounts than water without a thought as to their chemical content. Recently, a television viewer wrote to tell me that a friend of hers, a college student, was drinking three quarts of cola daily. That is equivalent to eight 12-oz. cokes containing 72 teaspoons of sugar (1-1/2 cups!) In addition to the sugar, there are from 240 to 464 mg. of caffeine, depending upon whose figures you believe!

Research has shown that 24 teaspoons of sugar eaten in one day reduces the number of bacteria that our white blood cells will destroy by 92 percent. I can't begin to guess what eating 300 percent more sugar would do to this young man's immune system. Research studies have convinced me that he can expect bone deterioration (including loose teeth in his jawbone), kidney stones, diabetes, heart disease, cancer, tooth decay, back problems, and a host of other illnesses.

In regard to the man's caffeine intake, a government booklet on the subject says we get a pharmacological or drug effect on a 60 to 100 mg. dose of caffeine. It continues to be reported that caffeine is associated with high levels of cholesterol which cause heart disease, and with low levels of the "good kind" of cholesterol that protects the heart from disease. Caffeine also encourages acquisition and natural development of peptic ulcers, diabetes, and hypoglycemia.

Research evidence also shows that caffeine causes an alteration in the chromosomes in the nuclei of cells and may be linked to cancer. I wonder what effect a daily intake of 300 to 400 percent *more* than a drug-effect dose would have on the body. I feel sure it is devastating to health, especially the heart and nervous system.

THE PEPSI GENERATION

Other facts about changes in our beverage consumption patterns are important to know. Whereas, in 1950, our thirsts were quenched predominantly by milk, water, and coffee, they are now satisfied by soft drinks, fruit drinks and "six packs" (beer).

In the amounts being consumed, the fruit drinks add too much sugar. In a sense, they too are addictive. Both soft drinks and beer contain addictive substances, and addiction leads to overconsumption. Overconsumption leads to obesity, one of the important at-risk factors for cancer, diabetes, heart disease, and a host of other degenerative diseases.

The addictive element in beer is, of course, alcohol. "Alcohol is itself a drug, sedative, tranquilizer, hypnotic, or anesthetic, depending on the quantity consumed."[4]

With the exception of beer, commonly consumed alcoholic beverages are devoid of nutrients. Beer has a small amount of thiamine, nicotinic acid, and protein; otherwise, all its calories are from alcohol. To make things even worse, regular drinking is known to affect food choices; irregular meals and ingestion of foods poor in nutrient density are the common patterns. This is often aggravated by gastritis, diminishing the beer drinker's appetite for normal foods.

As with heart disease, cancer, and diabetes, it takes years for the body to break down and permit disease to develop. The "Pepsi Generation" hasn't a ghost of a chance of escaping the kind of health problems that will remove them from the fun life in the fast lane!

IT'S UP TO YOU

Now that you know this information, how will you respond in regard to your eating habits? Hosea 4:6 says, "My people perish for a lack of knowledge."

While we need adequate, sound knowledge before making behavioral decisions, I sometimes think there is another problem at work when it comes to nutrition. People perish almost as often because they refuse to obey *known* facts. They know, for example, that fried and high-fat content foods (like most hamburgers) lead to disastrous heart problems. Still, they continue to eat regularly at fast-food restaurants and consume a daily diet high in fat.

They also know sugar "is supposed to be" bad for them, but how often do they reject sweet food solely on the basis that it has too much sugar in it for good health?

Which is worse, ignorance or disobedience? Our decision will determine whether we enjoy good health or suffer degenerative disease.

Many Americans are sick and need to change their thinking about the relationship between diet and health as well as diet and disease. What will you do?

NOW THE GOOD NEWS

After all this bad news, you will be glad to hear this good news: You are in charge of what you put into your own body.

In this book, and in my two earlier books, *Some Gold Nuggets in Nutrition* and *Are You Sick and Tired of Feeling Sick and Tired?*, you will find plenty of practical suggestions and a new way of looking at your eating habits. If you put them into practice, you will find that you can change.

And there is more good news: I have discovered a food concentrate that supplies the very nutritional elements in which the American diet has become deficient! This concentrate of vacuum-dried fresh juice of young green barley leaves (one teaspoon is equivalent to two handfuls of barley leaves) has the nutrient power to get you on your way to a healthier lifestyle.

It's as if our wise Creator put it together especially to cleanse and strengthen us while we make the basic nutritional changes in our eating and cooking habits. And, you know, I believe He did!

THE ANSWER TO OUR DILEMMA

One last word of advice. Do not have a cupboard and refrigerator "clean-out night" in which you discard all your "unhealthy" food. That only leads to total chaos and bilious (as well as rebellious) spirits!

Instead, establish the habit of making small improvements daily. Drink a few less soft drinks as you increase your daily consumption of pure water. Eat a healthful main dish some night for dinner instead of grilled pork chops with boxed au gratin potatoes. Forsake the doughnuts one morning in preference to shredded wheat topped with oat bran — and so forth. You will be surprised to see how easily you can improve your food intake by using this technique.

These new habits mean changing the way you shop for food. Planning menus would, of course, be the ideal way of assuring that you make changes and that you have the foods on hand to do so. If you can't get that organized, do it your way — but do it, and do it daily. It only takes 21 days of changed behavior to establish a "new" habit.

With the added help of the green leaves of barley — nature's miracle rejuvenator — you will be on your way to a new way of eating and living!

CHAPTER III

Barley — the Botanical Aristocrat

According to historians, barley is a well-known grain cultivated from the remotest antiquity.

Here are some facts about barley:

• It is the first grain to ripen in the spring; wheat is next and takes 4 to 6 weeks longer to mature.

• Because it is hardy and thrives in high altitudes and northern climatic conditions, barley is not attacked by bugs, molds, fungi, or worms, which abound later and in warmer climates.

• Barley is 67 percent carbohydrate and 12.8 percent protein —a "perfect" ratio of the two as claimed by modern scientists.

• Barley brought rejuvenation and renewal to the health of the ancient people whose winter diets were meager. It will do the same for us today.

• Regrettably, in America 54 percent is used in animal feed. Another large proportion goes into brewing beer and ale.

A NATURAL DEODORIZER

An M.D. who visited a farm family in Denmark one summer told me he had never forgotten the difference between Danish and American barns where cows were milked. Danish barns were absolutely odorless, even when fresh manure was on the straw-covered floor — but not so in American barns. The smell of manure was sometimes quite offensive.

When he asked the farmer about this observation, he was told that the reason was because of the barley in the cow's diet. "Barley is a natural deodorizer," he said.

A North Dakota farmer told me the same thing about the barley's deodorizing properties. Both barley grass and grain are filled with many enzymes. In addition, green barley is full of chlorophyll. Both aid in digestion and, when food is perfectly digested, waste from the intestinal tract is "clean" and odorless.

NATURE'S ANTACID

After I began to work on this book, I met a farmer from North Dakota who later wrote me a letter noting that barley straw is favored by cattle as a feed.

He also noted that on one area of his farm he had never been able to grow anything. When he planted it with barley, the ground produced approximately 70 bushels per acre!

Barley is considered a healer of the land. If the land is healed, isn't it logical to assume that it will produce healthy food, which will build healthy bodies or cause unhealthy bodies to rejuvenate themselves?

My farmer friend also noted that the "tied up" elements in the soil can be released by bringing the soil's pH to a preferred range.

Can this principle be applied to humans and the blood pH? Do all factors start doing their jobs properly by taking green barley (which is highly alkaline, as opposed to our acid-rich diet) to adjust our blood pH?

My answer to this is definitely, "Yes!" This is another illustration of how well integrated God has made everything He created. The soil pH affects the growth and health of all the plants just as the pH of the body fluids controls the digestion and assimilation of foods and the release and use of nutrients in humans and other animals.

The green leaves of embryonic barley plants are the most alkaline of any of the numerous green plants tested. For those who require an antacid after a meal in order to "feel good," a daily intake of a teaspoon or two of a pure green barley powder might very well eliminate the need for "artificial" preparations, which Americans are using at the cost of a half-billion dollars annually.

THE ABC'S OF GREEN BARLEY JUICE

The discovery of the amazing restorative power of the powdered juice of green barley leaves was born out of a personal tragedy. A Japanese medical doctor and research pharmacologist, Dr. Yoshihide Hagiwara, lost his health at the age of 38. He first tried to regain it by taking modern drugs and megadoses of synthetic vitamins and minerals, without success.

He then tried ancient Chinese herbal remedies and cleansing diets, with only slightly better results. When he sought healing in a diet rich in natural enzymes, raw chlorophyll, natural vitamins and minerals, and polypeptides (amino acids), he found it — the "physician within" brought back his health!

People today can attest to the effectiveness of eating raw, natural, unprocessed, organically grown food in the building, repair, and maintenance of healthy, disease-free cells in our bodies. Yes, when we remember our nutrition, we can usually forget disease!

GREEN BARLEY ESSENCE

Before Dr. Hagiwara selected barley leaves as his choice of "green foods" for product development, he spent ten years studying the roots, stems, twigs, leaves and flowers of more than 400 green plants—at all stages of maturity. (Read his book, *Green Barley Essence,* for full details.)

Finally, he found the *one* plant that was superior to all others. About it he wrote: "My research has shown that the green leaves of the embryonic barley plant contain the most prolific balanced supply of nutrients that exist on earth in a single source."[1]

After reading his book and studying his data, I am convinced that his powder of green barley leaves is indeed the prince of all green products. He found the right plant, the right growing methods, and developed and patented the right process for extracting and drying the juice. Because of the preparation method, most heat-sensitive components (proteins, including enzymes, as well as peptides and other components) remain in their natural state right along with heat-stable materials (minerals and polysaccharides).

After personally visiting his extensive research laboratories and his processing plant in Japan and California, I am convinced that his green barley product will always be unexcelled. I especially like the product he produces which has the addition of small amounts of powdered brown rice and kelp. These foods enhance the natural vitamin and mineral values lacking in our modern diet.

Although several other companies produce and market green barley products, I know of no other product resulting from the extensive and continuous scientific or medical research equivalent to Dr. Hagiwara's work in Japan. If there is another pharmacologically pure green barley product on the market, I have not found it.

In 1988, Dr. Hagiwara was honored by thousands of scientists and businessmen from all over the world, commemorating his 21 years of research and product development. It is little wonder that he has developed a food concentrate with such "power," considering the efforts put into the development of this food.

PURE EMERALD GREEN

Let me summarize the virtues of the dried barley juice I use as a daily supplement:

• The barley is grown organically, without artificial chemical fertilizers.

• No chemical sprays (pesticides, fungicides, herbicides) are used on the plants.

• The processing plant is "on site" so that the barley is harvested and processed with a very short time lapse.

• The special drying process sprays the juice in a vacuum at about 97° F for 2 to 3 seconds without subjecting the nutrients to destructive processing methods. Not even the enzymes are destroyed.

• It is immediately refrigerated until it can be bottled and kept as fresh and near "natural" as possible.

• When dissolved in anything cold to drink, it reconstitutes itself to be substantially the same as fresh raw juice.

• It is a powder similar in texture to instant coffee or tea (except for its emerald green color), and is just as easy to use (although the enzymes are destroyed if mixed with a hot liquid.)

• A teaspoonful (2 gms.) contains approximately 6 calories and is equivalent to 100 gms. (two big handfuls) of young barley leaves. It is also available in caplet form. (I personally prefer the powder over the caplet.)

• Regarding its taste, the ads say it's like spinach or green tea, but to me it's closer to how the lawn smells after it's just been mowed! In V-8 or carrot juice, it's almost imperceptible. Fruit juices also mask its flavor, half pineapple and half orange is good.

THE POWER OF PLANT PROTEIN

Since the barley is harvested at an early stage, before the nutrients are concentrated in the heads of grain, it is still full of growth material and juvenile factors that are undoubtedly useful to our own cells and tissues.

Young barley leaves are an excellent source of all the essential amino acids. (From these the body can make all of the other amino acids.)

All proteins are not created equal! The body can use proteins in some foods better than those found in others. Proteins from plant sources are very easily digested and assimilated. Not all, however, contain the full range of amino acids required for growth, repair, and maintenance of tissue. Barley juice powder is not among that group — it contains them all.

Many Americans seem to have the wrong idea about protein. In their minds is the idea that we need *meat* to grow "big muscles" with "great strength" and "great endurance." This is not true. Plant proteins are excellent at achieving the above goals as long as they are properly combined and consumed at the same meal. For example, rice and beans make a protein that will achieve the same body functions as meat.

Many studies show vegetarian diets, which incorporate adequate amounts of grains, legumes, nuts, sprouts, etc., produce healthy people. A biblical story is a good one to illustrate this.

In Chapter 1 of Daniel, he and his three friends refused to eat the king's food. After three years of a vegetarian diet with only water to drink, the king said of these four youths: "And in matters requiring information and balanced judgment, the king found these young men's advice 10 times better than that of all the skilled magicians and wise astrologers in his realm" (Daniel 1:20, TLB).

In recent years, a California nine-year study compared Seventh-Day Adventists with the general meat-eating population of California. It showed Adventists significantly healthier in every test with less degenerative disease and more productivity in their work, etc.

Vegetable proteins are well utilized by the body and have the added advantage of adding no fat or cholesterol to the diet. That is another reason I am excited about powdered green barley.

NUTRIENT BOOSTERS

Very small amounts of powdered brown rice and kelp have been added to the green barley powder I use (but not to other products by Dr. Hagiwara) for two basic reasons. They contribute to an improvement in texture, which results in better shipping qualities as well as improved shelf life. The main advantage, however, is that these two foods fortify some essential elements in the American diet and complete the nutritional balance of the product.

Sea vegetables, such as kelp, are known as "collectors of energy and concentrators of nutrients . . . they contribute significantly to a solar-based world food-and-energy production system."[2]

"Kelp is one of the best sources of iodine; it is also rich in B-complex vitamins, vitamins D, E, and K, calcium and magnesium. It is beneficial in maintaining the health of the mucous membranes and in providing the nutritional support required to prevent such conditions as arthritis, constipation, nervous disorders, rheumatism, colds, and skin irritations."[3]

A third author spoke of kelp as being used by the Japanese to treat goiter (enlargement of the thyroid gland in the neck). He also said anyone taking thyroid medicine should consult with his/her doctor after taking powdered green barley leaves for a few weeks. You might need to take less, or do away with your prescription medicine altogether.[4]

WHAT IT WILL DO FOR YOU

Green barley has certain amino acids which act as a gentle stimulant to the mucous membranes and lymphatic system and has long been recognized as a guardian against high blood pressure, especially among the elderly.

By promoting the balanced absorption and distribution of nutrients in the body, it is also beneficial to overweight and underweight people by helping to restore their normal weight conditions.

My own experience with those regularly taking this product is that many have experienced a normalizing of their weight and also a lowering of blood pressure. Kelp might be one of the contributing ingredients that brings health to the cells and, therefore, relief of symptoms in these two conditions.

Brown rice contains generous amounts of a number of vitamins and minerals. While the measure of brown rice in this food is small, it augments our supply of vitamin A, E, B_1, B_2, B_6, B_{12}, biotin, niacin, pantothenic acid, folic acid, plus the minerals of calcium, copper, iron, magnesium, manganese, phosphorus, potassium, selenium, sodium, and zinc.[5]

The green leaves of barley product is a food with real power.

TWO WHO RECOMMEND BARLEY WATER

Author Joseph Kadans writes that barley is mild and nutritional enough to help those with stomach ulcers and diarrhea. He also believes it helps prevent loss of hair and improves the condition of the nails of both hands and feet.

According to Mr. Kadans, barley water has been beneficial to those with gravel stones and high fever. He feels it may be useful in asthma because of a substance in the grain, hordenine, which relieves bronchial spasms.

To prepare a good barley drink, Mr. Kadans recommends taking 2 oz. of whole-grain barley and boiling it in three parts of water until the quantity of water is reduced by one half. The liquid remaining is considered good for bowel disorders, especially if 2 oz. of sliced figs are added during the cooking.[6]

Nelson Coons writes that some believe barley water is a "first food" for feeding infants who have kidney and bladder disorders. Mixed with lemon, barley water is an excellent drink for those suffering from bronchitis, asthma, and sore throat.[7]

While these ideas do not call for the use of barley juice, I included them here to show that the barley grain is also a valuable food for health. In fact, Hippocrates said, "Concerning nourishment, I think barley gruel is better than all other cereal foods in taking care of acute diseases; the finest barley should be used."[8]

This background on barley is provided to give a perspective on the real contribution barley grain has made through the ages to the health of all living creatures, including man.

THE SUPER GRAIN

In 1990, a study by Montana State University compared people who ate a diet high in barley with those who ate a lot of wheat products. The results showed some of the barley eaters experienced drops in cholesterol of up to 15 percent after four weeks. By contrast, the wheat eaters had either the same or higher cholesterol levels at the end of the study.

It was postulated that the fiber in barley (beta-glucans) was responsible for the lower cholesterol blood levels. Oats and barley contain significant amounts of this fiber, but wheat does not.

Tests done by the same researcher, Rosemary Newman, on laboratory animals indicated that another substance in barley, (an oil called tocotrienol, which is related to vitamin E), also plays a role in reducing cholesterol.

Hopefully this research will serve as a spring board for further study of the nutritional benefits of barley — making it the super aristocrat of the grain family.

CHAPTER IV

HEALTHY CELLS —
HEALTHY BODY

If all scientists in the world could agree on a single fact, I believe they would agree on this, "Life begins, is maintained and ends at the cellular level." The health of single cells holds the key to the health of the whole organism.

Why is this? Because single cells clump together to form tissues and tissues cluster to form organs. Thus, to keep individual cells healthy is to experience health in the whole body. In reverse, when individual cells become unhealthy, tissues can become unhealthy, and if unchecked, disease can result in the death of the whole person.

CELLS, TISSUES, ORGANS

1. Cells. A typical cell has two major parts — the nucleus and the cytoplasm.

Cytoplasm is composed of carbohydrates, proteins, fats, ions, and small compounds that differ from cell type to cell type. The nucleus of the cell is the "control center," which contains the coded information for the manufacture of all building blocks and enzymes.

2. Tissues. Cells of a similar type that are grouped together are called tissues.

Tissues of one kind depend upon other kinds of tissues to supply some of their needs to carry out their specific functions. An example of this interdependence of tissues can be illustrated by muscles whose primary function is movement.

Muscles cannot move without oxygen supplied by the blood tissue. Neither can they move without food from the digestive tract, which in itself is a complex system of various tissues. Muscles also require regulation of movement in both type and amount, which is provided by the tissues of the nervous system. The body furnishes us many illustrations of the interdependence of cells and tissues such as this one.

3. Organs, like the stomach, are simply groups of tissues joined together to perform specific tasks. The stomach lining is one kind of tissue, and the stomach muscles that cause the food to be thoroughly mixed are another kind, and so on.

DYNAMIC CELLS

Cells are the basic units of life and they are responsible for all the functions of living matter. Their duties are very specific, but when they are considered collectively, all the functions of the organism are perfectly met when the cells are healthy.

What determines the health status of individual cells? The ability of the cells to carry out their full range of functions. These are:

• **Enzymatic breakdown** of foods to provide more than 40 known nutrients for the building, repair, and maintenance of tissue, and for energy.

• **Absorption** of dissolved substances into cells to serve the same functions as listed above.

• **Synthesis,** or putting together of organic compounds from smaller units obtained from digestion and absorption or some other synthesis reaction in the cell. This results in the functions of cell growth, secretion, and replacement of worn-out cellular parts.

• **Cell respiration** which results in the release of energy from the final stage of the digestion of food.

• **Cell movement** and the movement of substances inside the cell which determine its efficiency in functioning.

• **Excretion** of waste products (toxins and the "clinkers" of metabolism) from cells. Some waste materials to be removed are soluble, others are nonsoluble and nondigestible.

• **Homeostasis,** which means to maintain a steady state within a cell and permits its existence and formation of new cells.[1]

Every cell works constantly in this "dynamic equilibrium" state of existence. Once there is too great a change in the set of conditions required for functioning, the cell dies and the organism can lose its equilibrium and also die. Homeostasis cannot be maintained under unfavorable cell conditions.

Let's look at how certain factors affect the internal and external structure of the cell.

WHAT A HEALTHY CELL NEEDS

1. The Internal Temperature. The cell functions normally within a narrow range of temperature — around 98.6°F. If the body temperature may falls lower than 77°F., cell damage will take place and medical treatment will be required.[2]

When the body temperature rises above 104°-106°F., cells begin to be damaged or destroyed throughout the whole body, especially in the brain where, unfortunately, they cannot be replaced. Organs are also damaged during periods of extremely high fever — the liver and kidneys especially. This damage can be severe enough to cause death. That is why it is necessary to keep a person's body temperature below 104°F. during a time of illness.[3]

2. The Acid-Base Balance — pH. Cells function best when the pH is within the rather narrow range of 7.35 to 7.45. Enzymes within the cell are also affected by pH. A highly acid or highly alkaline cell environment will cause an improper functioning or a total cessation of functioning.

3. The Absence of Chemical Substances. All prescription drugs (chemicals) are toxic and have multiple, negative side effects. All create cell stress and the need for the type of healing that only nature can provide.

Consider some of the negative effects of drinking alcohol:
- Causes the cells of the mouth and throat to dehydrate and become numb.
- Irritates and inflames the esophagus cells, the stomach, and the duodenum, the lungs and the liver.
- Interferes with normal functioning of the nerves.
- Poisons the cells of the respiratory system and liver.
- Poisons brain cells, causing them to malfunction, atrophy, or die.[4]

4. Pure Water. The fluid nature of water enables both dissolved and suspended substances to move or flow within the cell. When inadequate amounts of water are consumed, negative effects results, such as:
- The action of electrolytes (minerals and charged particles) is hindered.
- Production and functioning of hormones is adversely affected.
- Digestion of food is stymied.

Cells are dependent upon the extracellular fluid around them to carry oxygen from the lungs to the tissues and to remove the carbon dioxide. This fluid is in constant motion and rapidly mixed by the blood circulation flowing past the cells for maintenance of cellular function. A number of pathological conditions obstruct this blood flow and interfere with cell health.

Some of these are: removal of lung tissue, blood clots in the lung, traumatized fatty tissue clogging the lungs (as is often the case in breast surgery), emphysema, collapse of a lung, etc. When blood flow is decreased and the oxygen supply to the cell is diminished, the cells cannot receive either nourishment or oxygen and death is the end result.

Cells are perfectly capable of living, growing, reproducing, and performing their special functions only so long as blood, muscles, organs, glands, and body fluids bring them the proper concentrations of oxygen, glucose, vitamins, minerals, amino acids, and fatty substances required by our body's internal environment.

GRASS, HERBS, AND TREES

On the third day of creation, God said, "Let the earth bring forth grass, the herb yielding seed . . . And then God saw that it was good" (Genesis 1:11, 12).

On the sixth day of creation, God created man and woman and said, "Behold I have given you every herb bearing seed, which is given upon the face of all the earth, and every tree, in which is the fruit of a tree yielding seed; to you it shall be for meat" (Genesis 1: 29). Webster's dictionary lists as the first definition of meat, "food, especially food, as distinguished from drink."

In this verse, three distinct types of vegetation are mentioned — grass, herbs, and trees. Someday scientists will prove that these three kinds of vegetation, along with pure air, pure water, enough rest, and proper exercise will hold the key to as perfect health as possible on this planet.

God created a magnificent human body and then provided perfectly for its growth, maintenance, and repair of tissue (healing), without any opportunity for a physical or chemical conflict.

God put upon this earth every ingredient needed to promote and sustain cell life. In addition, I believe He also put on this earth the stems, roots, leaves, and bark containing every ingredient necessary to change a sick cell to a healthy cell.

DNA and RNA were designed by God to tell each healthy cell how to reproduce itself, to energize itself, to empty itself of waste, and to heal itself when attacked by "foreigners."

If cells are given the proper ingredients in the right amounts at the right time, they will reproduce themselves and live in health without the use of any outside substance. A Nobel Prize was given to the scientist who proved this point by keeping a chicken heart alive in a test-tube for years and years, just by providing it with nature's cell recipe and removing the toxins that were given off by it as it used the nutrients.

Adam and Eve were supplied with an abundance of whole, natural, pure, fresh, ready-to-eat, delicious foods — the exact substances needed for healthy cells. The supplies of fruits, vegetables, whole grains, legumes, nuts, seeds, and berries were more than sufficient to sustain life in perfect chemical balance.

DEAD FOODS — DEAD BODIES

Let me illustrate how cells respond when fed the North American diet with its processed, refined, "artificial" and junk food.

Let's say that a brain cell corresponds to a biscuit recipe. It requires flour, shortening, salt, baking powder, and milk. Given high quality products in the right amounts with the right mixing techniques and baking methods, excellent biscuits (healthy cells) can result every time.

But think of it this way. Instead of shortening, we use axle grease; for flour, we substitute cement mix; we add a little gunpowder to replace the leavening agent; sand replaces the salt; some polluted liquid replaces nature's pure, raw, fresh-from-the-cow milk.

What happens to the brain cells? Is it any wonder that we have tumors, cancers, aneurysms, Alzheimer's disease, and a host of other conditions related to not having the right ingredients in the brain cell recipe?

Multiply this nutritional travesty three times a day, most days and weeks of the year, and it is easy to see how our poor quality foods are negatively impacting the health of our cells.

Cells are perfectly capable of living, growing, reproducing, healing themselves, and performing special functions only so long as the blood, muscles, organs, glands, and body fluids bring them the proper concentrations of vitamins, minerals, amino acids, fatty substances, oxygen, and glucose required by our bodies' internal environment.

All of the functions of our bodies depend upon the health of our organs. The health of our organs depends upon the health of the tissues that comprise the organs. The health of the tissues depends on healthy individual cells. The health of the cells depends upon the supply of nutrients and oxygen and liquid in the blood. The supply of nutrients in the blood depends upon the foods we eat.

Natural foods are the most perfect sources of all the nutrients needed or required for health. **Lifeless cells make lifeless people just as surely as "dead foods" make dead people.**

What is the source of health? It is our marvelous, self-restoring, self-healing, aggregate of 75 to 83 trillion cells, aided by a sound mind and healthy spirit. Neither medicine nor surgery, nor the absence of germs produces health. It is the proper functioning of every part of the body, with adequate amounts of pure air, pure water, healthy food, exercise, and a strong immune system, to mention a few.

KEEPING YOUR CELLS HEALTHY

The typical North American diet definitely needs improvement. To keep your cells healthy, I recommend:

• A teaspoon or two of the powdered juice of green barley leaves daily. It is one of the most nutrient-dense foods you can buy to provide cells with elements crucial to their optimal functioning.

• Omit toxic foods such as soft drinks, tea, coffee, spices, chocolate, foods that contain preservatives, foods that are dyed, waxed, sprayed with chemicals, etc.

• Eliminate white sugar and white flour.

Cells always respond to an improvement in the quality of your diet. Regardless of the extent or length of time you have had sick cells, they will make a herculean effort to improve when given the right nutrients. Our bodies are programmed for health, not illness. I hope you will begin to try a little harder to cooperate with nature's plan for using sound nutrition principles to achieve robust health.

CREATING A CYCLE OF WELL-BEING

A positive mental attitude is absolutely crucial to the concept of healthy cells. There is a constant interplay between our mental and bodily reactions. "Many nervous and emotional disturbances, high blood pressure, arthritis, gastric and duodenal ulcers, cancer, and certain types of sexual, allergic, cardiovascular, and kidney malfunctions appear to be essentially diseases of adaptation."[5]

In the absence of learning to adapt to these life situations, we succumb to innumerable illnesses and diseases.

Poor health may start with a clogged up metabolism, with its resulting low energy level. Is low energy a "symptom" of depression, drug abuse, etc.? Or is it the cause? Good nutrition has tremendous potential in these areas because it simply, demonstrably, can change people's energy levels and outlooks for the better.

Dried green barley juice, a food rich in nutrients, can be used by the body to promote cell health and break the vicious cycle of depression.

If your cells are trying to live in a polluted environment, they cannot function properly to maintain the body/mind system at its peak. Besides nourishing brain cells and unclogging the metabolism that serves the brain, nutrients can actually boost your built-in pollution control mechanisms. In doing this, it can raise your energy level and produce an overall sense of well-being in body and mind.

As your sense of well-being increases, your mind begins to produce more optimistic forecasts, which can be self-fulfilling and self-reinforcing. As your mental attitude becomes more positive, you are more likely to seek out and engage in what is good for you. This is the way to a cycle of ever-increasing well-being.

EXERCISING TOXINS AWAY

Have you ever given thought to how your body rids itself of cell waste — called "toxins"? Would you be surprised if I told you it requires exercise for efficient removal of these products? Without the removal of toxins from the cells, we would die within 24 hours.[6]

Almost all tissues of the body (you remember, tissues are simply structures made from similar cells to perform a specific purpose) drain excess fluid directly from the spaces between cells. If there were not a system provided for clearing this interstitial fluid, there would be "system-wide" swelling that would probably eventually lead to death.

We often see swelling at the ankles, under the eyes, and in other tissues. But nature, of course, knew that would happen before we did, so the perfect provision for elimination of all waste has been made. The route provided is called the lymphatic system and the fluid removed is called lymph. The lymph contains plasma proteins and large particles of matter, neither of which are able to be removed by the blood.

Bacteria, viruses, and other foreign matter are also filtered out and destroyed. This is done by a pumping action of the muscle fibers (a form of exercise) in the lymph vessel walls. The lymph is moved upward, never backward, by the pressure of skeletal muscle contraction as you move your body. So, there we have it — cell health through exercise.[7]

A few minutes a day on a trampoline, or a minimum of 30 minutes of very brisk walking, greatly stimulate the lymph nodes throughout the body to filter debris before they return to the bloodstream.

People who are "active," whether or not they have a specific exercise program, get rid of more cell debris (toxins) than those who live sedentary lives. Therefore, if you are one who is always tired and lacks real zest for living, exercise the toxins out of your cells and "feel the difference."

YOUR CELLS' DEFENSE SYSTEM

The body's defense system has protected man for centuries from being annihilated in an unfriendly environment filled with many types of pathogenic (disease-producing) organisms. In addition, modern man is assaulted daily by impure water, impure air, chemically polluted soil, and a food chain filled with all kinds of cell health enemies. How have we been able to survive?

In the first place, we were born with some very basic systems of protection — an army, a navy, and an air force of sorts.

THE ARMY

1. The Skin. This major organ serves as the first line of defense against bacteria, viruses, and many organisms and chemicals that could be very harmful to our system, were they permitted to enter.

The skin doesn't even allow significant amounts of harmless substances, like water or air, to get inside. It is an effective cell protector. In addition, the skin produces small amounts of vitamin D and the male sex hormone, testosterone. The skin also excretes a small amount of waste from the cells in the form of sweat. So, this is a highly valuable form of health defense.

2. *Mucous Membranes*. These line the digestive, respiratory, urinary, and reproductive tracts. The mucous secreted by these protective membranes forms a wall around invaders that would destroy health, traps the offenders, and then destroys them. The mucus in the nose, for example, filters "tons" of potentially harmful substances and holds them trapped by the cilia (hair-like projections), and we are able to blow these from the nose passages. If they are swallowed instead, as sometimes is the case, the highly acidic juice of the stomach effectively puts any pathogens out of commission — forever.

3. *Friendly Bacteria*. These live in our intestines and produce some valuable protectors of cell health — the B-vitamins. These intestinal flora, as they are called, are still a mystery to medical science, but their beneficial qualities are neither doubted nor denied by them. What doctors often ignore is the fact that prescription drugs, which they so freely dispense, are destroyers of these wonderful defenders. When the protection of the intestinal flora is lost, it is easy for the pathogenic bacteria to replace them in the gut and we can so easily become ill with disease. (Think about that when you so thoughtlessly swallow synthetic drugs!)

4. *Tear Glands*. These keep the eyeballs moist and free from air pollutants as well as providing us the blessing of tears. Tears contain an enzyme which attacks the cell walls of bacteria and protects the eyes from invasion by these harmful enemies of the cells. Any person who has experienced "dry eyes" fully understands the benefits to eyeball cells when there is moisture present.

THE NAVY

If some of our enemies were clever enough to avoid death at the hand of our army's tactics, the second line of defense is right there, ready for quick action. The navy's arsenal of weapons is composed of:

1. A higher-than-normal temperature (fever).
2. The lymphatic system
3. Phagocytes — a special kind of fighter cells.

We have already discussed temperature and the lymphatic system. Phagocytes will be covered separately in the chapter on the immune system. This navy, however, is an important part of our cell defense system, and we couldn't have healthy cells without it.

THE AIR FORCE

This defense system is made up of chemicals — complex protein molecules made by the body and called antibodies. Carried from place to place in the body by the blood, they can destroy the toxins produced by certain pathogens and can even destroy the pathogens themselves. These microorganisms are called antigens, and the antibodies are produced by our air force in the thymus gland, the spleen, and the lymph nodes. More about this will be discussed under the subject of immunity in an upcoming chapter.

THE BODY: A SELF-RESTORING SYSTEM

If you are in good health and want to stay that way, or if you are ill and want to get well, success in either of these situations depends largely upon you — no one else can do it for you!

How does the body protect and repair itself, rejuvenate and rebuild tissues torn down through wear and tear of daily living? By using the same chemical elements from which it was made — minerals, vitamins, enzymes, protein, carbohydrates, fats, and water. I do not believe good health is accomplished through drugs and man-made concoctions containing specific amounts and types of unnatural elements. Nothing man can put together in the way of magic formulas for health will ever heal or rebuild or promote growth like the products provided for us by nature.

Nature cures; nature heals; nature grows new cells, new blood, new bones, new tissues, and all the rest. It works slowly and tediously, taking its time whether we like it or not. But, it works to perfection. Perfection is its goal. It just needs our cooperation in being positive, and patient! We must believe it is working, and that recovery is on the way.

Chapter V

Your Personal "Star Wars"

by Susan C. Darbro
BA in English, BS in Nursing

In the last 10 years, an explosion of new information has surfaced, bringing with it a new and deeper understanding of what the immune system is and how it works. Your immune system is what protects you from invasion and infection. That is why I call it your personal "Star Wars."

THE INVADERS

The immune system protects the body from invasion, but how does the immune system know who and what is the enemy?

The body has the ability to recognize its own parts as "self" and other things as "nonself." Invaders are nonself, and are usually referred to by the term *antigen(s)*. An antigen can be a virus, a bacterium, a fungus, or a parasite, or even a portion or product of one of these organisms.

Tissues or cells from another individual, unless it is an identical twin, can also act as antigens. Because a transplanted organ is seen as "foreign," the body's natural response is to reject it.

The body will even reject nourishing proteins unless they are first broken down, by the digestive system, into their primary building blocks.[1] Antigens such as viruses, bacteria, and fungi must penetrate healthy cells in order to reproduce. That is their goal, and that is what the immune system seeks to prevent.

When we fail to take good care of our bodies by neglecting to practice good health habits — proper diet, adequate rest, and regular exercise — we risk an invasion. To have strong and healthy immune systems, we need strong, healthy bodies to house them in.

THE TRANSPORTATION NETWORK

Many organ systems in the body — like your urinary tract or digestive tract — are interconnected and function in a logical, progressive order just like the plumbing in a house. The immune system, however, is not like that. Different parts of it are found here, there, and everywhere in our bodies.

Immune system tissues are called "lymphoid tissues." They include the tonsils and adenoids in your neck, the thymus gland in your chest, the spleen in the left side of your abdomen, the appendix in the right side of your abdomen, the bone marrow inside the long bones of your body, the lymph nodes scattered throughout your body, and various blood and tissue cells which are almost everywhere at once.

Also included in this is your "lymphatic system" — a network of drainage vessels which parallels the bloodstream, vital to the functioning of the immune system. Like a system of small creeks and streams that empty into larger and larger rivers, the vessels of the lymphatic network merge into increasingly larger tributaries. At the base of the neck, the large lymphatic ducts empty into the bloodstream.[2]

THE LINE OF DEFENSE

Our bodies are specially constructed to resist disease, like a stone wall or high fence keeps strangers out of a house. Our first line of defense is our skin, which we can think of as a protective coating or shell for our body. It is specially equipped with secretions of fatty acids that have a deadly effect on certain microorganisms.[3] Unless we damage it by some kind of injury, it is sufficient to keep most would-be invaders out.

The size of the invader is of little importance because tiny invaders can be just as deadly as those we can see. The AIDS virus, for example, is so small that 230 million of them could fit in a space no bigger than the period at the end of this sentence.[4] A tiny scratch or pinprick can have fatal consequences, and it is important for you to keep wounds clean and covered, particularly when you are around someone who is sick.

Another one of the custom-made features we have at our disposal is in the respiratory tract. Here tiny hair-like projections lining the respiratory tract trap foreign bodies and prevent them from lodging inside cells, where they can begin to grow and multiply.

In addition, special linings of our respiratory and digestive tracts called mucous membranes ooze out a thick, sticky substance which also traps invaders. Special enzymes found in tears and saliva are harmful to many organisms, just in case we get some in our eyes or mouth. Many body fluids, including blood, also contain chemical substances to counteract an attack by antigens.

GOBBLING UP INVADERS

The macrophage is a large, specialized cell, whose job it is to engulf and consume foreign substances. A macrophage is one type of phagocyte, which engulfs and digests invaders.

If we get caught sitting next to someone who sneezes, a macrophage in our body comes along and sees that the sneezed particles are "nonself" and immediately tries to consume them before they can reach the safety of the interior of a cell. (That is assuming those hair-like projections failed to trap the particles in the nose and windpipe.)

Phagocytes are an extremely important part of our immune system.

GOING ON THE ATTACK

Stem cells produce baby fighter cells that travel to other parts of the body to mature. If they mature in bone marrow, they become "B cells;" whereas, if they go through the thymus gland, they become

"T cells." Stem cells do not themselves participate directly in an immune attack, but they produce the fighter cells which do.

The immune defense system is often divided into two categories, something like the army and the navy. One part is called "humoral." The other division is called cellular or "cell-mediated."

There are several types of T cells (technically, they are "T lymphocytes"):

1. *Helper T Cell* — turns T cells and B cells on.

2. *Suppressor T Cell* — calls off the fight after an immune response has successfully repelled an invasion.

3. *Natural Killer Cell* — attacks and destroys other cells by puncturing their cell membranes. Killer cells will attack our own body cells if they have been taken over by antigens. Killer cells prowl around our bodies looking for abnormalities, like cancer cells, and destroy them.

Many more kinds of T lymphocytes exist in the ranks of our immune system, but these three represent the major types of fighter cells.

AN ARSENAL OF WEAPONS

B cells (actually B lymphocytes) are born of a mother stem cell and then mature in bone marrow. The main job of a B cell is to secrete substances called antibodies. Antibodies are like snowflakes or fingerprints in that each one is different and made for one specific antigen.

Millions of antigens exist, and our body has the capacity to make antibodies to fit each one, just as a key fits in a lock. "By storing just a few cells specific for each potential invader, it (our body) has room for the entire army."[5] Thus, "The immune system stockpiles a tremendous arsenal."[6]

When an antigen appears, the B cell that matches it swells into what is called a "plasma cell" and begins to rapidly reproduce antibodies. Many B cells are unable to recognize the foreign body until a macrophage displays partially digested antigen on its surface.

Antibodies do not all function alike. Some cause invaders to dissolve. Others change the surface of the antigens so they clump together, making it impossible for them to function. Clumping also makes it easier for macrophages and other scavenger cells to find and digest them. Other antibodies coat the antigens to make them attractive to phagocytes. Still others cover them with poisonous protein which renders the antigens harmless. Some surround an area and cordon it off.

T memory cells and B memory cells have "photographic" memories of invaders and can program the body to make antibodies against them at the drop of a hat. Memory cells live for years. That is why a child who contracts measles at age two will never get them again, in spite of the fact that he is exposed time and time again over the years.

THE WORST OFFENDERS
If you feed your body the right stuff, it will work for you, and if you don't, it won't. Some of our favorite foods literally paralyze our immune system. Let's look at the worst offenders:

1. Sugar. Researchers have discovered that sugar decreases our body's ability to destroy bacteria — it destroys our immune system![7] There are nine teaspoons of sugar in one 12-ounce Coke. This means if you drink three Cokes (or other soft drinks) in one day, you have immobilized 92 percent of your defense troops!

2. Lead, Cadmium, Mercury. According to Dr. Weiner, "Our food, water, and air have steadily become contaminated with the heavy metals — lead, cadmium, and mercury. In animal studies, these metals suppress all aspects of immune functions . . . and increasing susceptibility to infection." Cadmium is produced by cigarette smoke and organic fertilizers made from sewage sludge. "Elevated cadmium levels have been shown to depress bone marrow function."[8]

3. Dietary Fat. High dietary fat intake can seriously impair immune functioning[9] and high dietary cholesterol may diminish cell-mediated and humoral immunity.[10]

"A high-fat diet leads to elevated levels of bile acids in the colon. These break down into deoxycholic acids, which are dangerous carcinogens . . . cancer of the breast, pancreas, gallbladder, ovary, uterus and prostate, as well as leukemia, are all positively correlated with a diet high in animal protein fat and cholesterol . . . High-fat diets and obesity also correlate strongly with the incidence, tumor size and speed of development of breast cancer."[11]

IMMUNE SYSTEM SUPPORT

How can we help our immune system? One way is to take barley juice daily because it contains the nutrients needed to support our immune system. Let's look at some of the most important vitamins and minerals contained in barley juice:

1. Vitamin A. Barley juice is a good source of vitamin A. What does Vitamin do for our bodies?

• Preserves the integrity of skin and mucous membranes
• Helps maintain the protective barriers against infectious organisms entering the body
• Needed for the production of bacteria-fighting lysozymes in tears, saliva and sweat [12]
• Enhances resistance to infection[13]

2. Vitamin B_1. When this vitamin is deficient in the diet, the size of lymphatic organs grows smaller and the number of T and B cells decreases.[14] Barley juice is a wonderful source of this important nutrient.

3. Vitamin B_2. Called riboflavin, the vitamin is found in large amounts in barley juice. Riboflavin is an immunity promoter and is involved in the production of antibodies.

4. Vitamin B_6. Also called pyridoxine, it is plentiful in barley juice, and "seems to be the most important for proper immune functioning with deficiencies causing more serious immune problems than with the other B vitamins.[15] Researchers found that "volunteers with short-term experimental B_6 deficiencies could not react properly to vaccines."[16]

5. Vitamin B$_{12}$. Cyanocobalamine is essential for the formation of red blood cells. It is also needed to treat defectively formed red blood cells.

6. Folic Acid. Folic acid deficiency depresses immune functions[17] and causes the body to let tumors grow more easily.[18] Barley juice is high in folic acid!

7. Choline. Without this nutrient, which is found in barley juice, the humoral immune division does not function properly. This is especially true when dietary lack occurs during pregnancy.[19]

8. Vitamin C. Researchers tell us that besides helping the phagocytes get from where they are to where they are needed, vitamin C also influences the killing functions of fighter cells. You should also note that aspirin has an anti-vitamin C effect, "promoting the loss of vitamin C through the urine and also decreasing uptake of the vitamin by white blood cells. Taking aspirin also seems to increase the danger of a spreading viral infection . . . For these reasons, you may want to think twice before taking aspirin along with vitamin C for your cold or flu."[20]

9. Copper. Minerals, like copper, are also necessary for the proper functioning of our immune system. "Copper deficiency has been linked to lower resistance."[21] Barley juice is a good source of copper.

10. Iron. Also contained in barley juice, this mineral is necessary to get oxygen to the cells, and the cells of the immune system have a "relatively high" oxygen requirement.[22] Caution, however, should be used in taking iron supplements because too much iron is just as dangerous to our bodies as not enough.

11. Zinc. Abundant in barley juice, this mineral "is an extremely important immune stimulant, specifically promoting T cell immunity"[23] Without zinc, the activity of killer cells is lower, antibodies do not function well, and the growth of stem cells in the thymus gland is adversely affected.[24]

Did you know that vitamin D, which our bodies make themselves, can actually suppress immune functioning? Guess what — barley juice doesn't have any!

Of course, any fat-soluble vitamin can build up in the body and cause problems if you take too much over a long period of time. So, be careful with your supplements, particularly if you are faithful in taking dried barley juice.

If we want to keep healthy, we must keep our immune system functioning in tip-top condition. Barley juice is full of vitamins and minerals that the immune system needs. One of the best ways we can help ourselves remain free of disease is to drink dried barley juice on a regular basis.

CHAPTER VI

Chlorophyll: A Wonder Drug?

by Susan C. Darbro
BA in English, BS in Nursing

To appreciate the power barley juice has to improve your health, you must understand a little about chlorophyll, and in order to understand chlorophyll, we need to review photosynthesis.

What gives barley juice its green color? Chlorophyll, a pigment found in all plants. It manifests itself in different but chemically related groups: chlorophyll-a, chlorophyll-b, etc. The majority of chlorophyll is in the form of chlorophyll-a, found in all "oxygen evolving" organisms.

As you know, plants do not eat eggs for breakfast, or lunch at McDonald's in order to get food for energy. They must make their own sugars and starches using only air, water, and sunshine. The recipe is quite long and involved, and our friend chlorophyll is a major ingredient.

Chlorophyll molecules act as tiny but powerful antennae to absorb light and transfer it to other chlorophyll molecules which undergo chemical oxidation, converting light into chemical energy the plant can use.

Photosynthesis is the process by which the plant takes carbon dioxide from the air, water from the soil, and light energy from the sun and puts them all together to use for its growth and maintenance. The important thing to remember is that photosynthesis would be impossible without chlorophyll.

This makes chlorophyll a very important substance to you and me. If there were no chlorophyll, there would be no photosynthesis. If there were no photosynthesis, there would be no plant life. Without plants, there could be no animal life on earth, including us! Chlorophyll, therefore, is absolutely essential to life.

THE "BLOOD" OF PLANTS

Scientific research on chlorophyll in the arena of medicine involves mostly two types. One is chlorophyll-a, which is chemically structured so that it doesn't dissolve in water. Early researchers believed that the chlorophyll found in nature, therefore, was of little practical use.

Newer research, however, substantiates the fact that raw, naturally occurring chlorophyll is absorbed in the intestines, following the same pathway that digestion of vitamin A takes.[1] Natural chlorophyll would be much better absorbed were it not encased in plant fiber. One advantage green barley powder has over fresh vegetables in this regard is that, because its fiber is removed, its chlorophyll is very easily digested. Both naturally occurring chlorophyll and its chlorophyllin derivatives have immense therapeutic value.

The green pigment in plants and the red pigment in blood are nearly identical. The major difference is that the central atom in chlorophyll is magnesium, whereas the central atom in hemoglobin is iron. What is the significance? The pigment chlorophyll is the "blood" of plants, and the fact it bears such a striking resemblance to the oxygen carrying pigment coloring our blood is no idle curiosity.

One of the first to see this connection was Dr. Hans Fischer, who used it in the treatment of anemic patients.[2] Researchers saw that the similarity between chlorophyll and hemoglobin went one step further — both remained nearly identical during breakdown processes. When partly digested grass was fed to rats, "it directly stimulated formation of red blood cells."[3]

Scientists admit that the blood of humans and animals and the chlorophyll in plants is "similar in all biological systems."[4]

CHLOROPHYLL THE HEALER

Dr. Benjamin Gruskin found that chlorophyll has a "stimulating effect upon the growth of supportive connective tissue cells and development of granulation tissue."[5] This has enormous significance in medicine, especially in the field of surgery, because the body must repair itself and chlorophyll helps it to do so.

"Granulation tissue" is the early, grainy cells which appear on the surface of wounds during healing. Chlorophyll speeds up the process! The application of chlorophyllins increases local blood supply.[6] Since blood supplies the nutrients and oxygen cells need to reproduce, greater blood supply means greater healing power.

Another reason for the acceleration of the healing process is that, when a wound becomes inflamed, the red blood cells become clumped together and are, therefore, unable to work efficiently. Chlorophyll has an "inhibitory effect" on clumping.[7]

Chlorophyll in ointment form has also been used in the treatment of various skin conditions and chronic ulcers. Ear, nose, and throat specialists used chlorophyll on patients with chronic sinus infections, resulting in "a final cure of all former symptoms."[8]

A WONDER DRUG?

Dr. Gruskin and associates treated a whole host of conditions, including open wounds, infections in deep surgical wounds, fistulas (abnormal drainage tracts communicating within the body) of the abdomen and chest, emphysema (pus in the lungs), abscesses of the liver and kidney, rectal lesions, leg ulcers due to poor circulation, brain abscesses, gangrenous appendicitis, and uterine cancer. He says, "From this partial list of cases, it becomes apparent the use of chlorophyll in any acute or chronic suppurative (containing pus) process has resulted in definite improvement."[9]

Chlorophyll has the ability to break down carbon dioxide and release oxygen, which spells disaster for many bacteria that thrive in deep wounds away from air.

Studies by other medical researchers found that:

• "Chlorophyll" tablets deodorized patients with colostomies (artificial openings in the lower intestine near the rectum) and enabled them to resume normal lives.

• Chlorophyllin dressings deodorized and speeded the healing of stubborn osteomyelitic bone infections and prompt healing in a wide variety of mouth infections.

• Chlorophyllin preparations were the most effective in healing bed sores and severe burns.[10]

• During World War II, chlorophyll therapy was responsible for saving the limbs of several wounded soldiers from amputation.[11]

• In a study of female patients in a geriatric nursing home, chlorophyllin successfully controlled body and fecal odors in 85 percent and helped combat constipation as well as relieved gas discomfort in 50 percent of those same patients whose bowel difficulties were otherwise not readily manageable.[12]

• One report notes, "There seems to be a trend for chlorophyllin efficacy in decreasing urinary odor."[13]

• Soluble chlorophyllin both retards the growth of crystals (kidney "stones" are really crystals) and prolongs the time it takes for them to get started.[14]

Chlorophyll is just as much a "wonder drug" as the man-made wonder drugs of this century. And barley green juice is packed full of this easily digested chlorophyll.

CHAPTER VII

End of the Acid Stomach

In describing the outstanding qualities of barley leaves as a food with real power, the fact that it is highly alkaline is a great advantage for those eating a typical American "high acid-ash" diet. To understand this, you need to understand the symbol pH.

What does pH mean and why is it important? The pH is the measurement of the ratio between acids and alkalines in our body fluids — ranging from 0 to 14.0 with neutral being 7.0. Acid is from 0 to 7.0 and alkaline 7.0 to 14.0.

A list of the pH of some of the most important substances would include the following:[1]

Acid:	Stomach Acid (HCl)........1.0	Urine..........................6.0
	Gastric Acid....................1.4	
Neutral:	Pure Water.....................7.0	
Alkaline:	Blood..............................7.35	Bile..............................7.5
	Pancreatic Juice.............8.5	

A quick way to determine a person's pH balance is to check the pH of his urine. From the above list, you can see that if a person's urine pH, for example, is on the acid side, the pH is expressed as a lower number on the pH scale than if it is normal.

The opposite is true of alkaline urine. It would be expressed by a number higher than average and the doctor would say you have a higher than normal pH. One of the keys to vibrant health, therefore, is keeping your pH in balance.

WATER AND A BALANCED pH

A high urine pH usually indicates the person is not drinking enough water. Few Americans, I am told, drink adequate amounts of water — not liquids but water — for good health. Our gallons of soft drinks, iced tea, and instant beverage mixes don't count.

Your weight in pounds divided by two is the correct number of ounces of water needed daily. If you're suffering from poor and/or slow digestion, low energy and a sluggish colon, your problem may be easily corrected by drinking more water!

The key to vibrant health is partly a matter of keeping your pH in balance. The cells in our body cannot function if the pH varies too far from the narrow range of 7.35 to 7.45. The maintenance of a constant pH ultimately depends upon the excretory action of the lungs and the kidneys.

ACID-BASE FORMING FOODS

After foods we eat are digested, they break down into either acid or an alkaline end-product in our tissues. This end-product is called the "ash" and remains in the body. Foods that produce an alkaline ash are "base-forming" foods, and those producing acid ash are called "acid-forming." These terms refer to the way the body uses our foods; it has nothing to do with the way they taste in your mouth.

A number of popular fruits, such as oranges, lemons, limes, cherries, grapefruit, etc., are sour and taste acid. Upon ingestion, however, they break down into a base-forming (alkaline) ash. This is a fact, but the average person, not understanding it, typically responds, "I don't care what anybody says, grapefruit is too acid for my system and I won't touch it."

Only prunes, plums, rhubarb, or cranberries burn leaving an acid ash and can accurately be claimed for making body fluids acid. If citrus fruit, for example, causes acidosis symptoms, it is because the citric acid has stirred up acid products already in the body for the purpose of detoxifying and eliminating them. This reaction may be uncomfortable, but is beneficial. If it happens to you, cut back on citrus for a few days and then resume eating small quantities occasionally until the problem passes.[2]

The body needs both types of foods. It is better, however, when alkaline (base-forming) foods slightly predominate over acid-forming ones. The body can handle a wide range of acid-base foods without upsetting the balance.

THE NORTH AMERICAN DIET

Today's North American diet, however, has pushed above this range of normalcy. We have become too full of acid and, as a result, are experiencing a wide range of diseases that flourish in an acid medium. That is one reason why dried barley juice is such an outstanding food — it is highly alkaline.

When you understand the foods that are in each of these two categories, it becomes very clear why our bodies are too acid in pH.

Acid-forming foods are: meat, fish, poultry, eggs, cereal products, corn, and sugars of all kinds.

Alkaline-forming foods are: milk, nuts, fruits, vegetables, and most seeds.[3]

Can you see why our American diet needs changing if we want to live a healthy and disease-free life?

CARBOHYDRATE SOURCES

Let's consider carbohydrate foods and their contribution to the pH balance in our bodies. Carbohydrates are of two major types — sugars and starches. Both of these groups leave an acid-ash upon digestion.

Sugars: Some of the major sources of sugar in the North American diet are: cane sugar, jellies, jams, fruit juices, preserves, soft drinks, dried fruits, candy, cake icing, etc. Hidden sugars like honey, molasses, syrups, beet sugar, lactose, corn syrup, glucose, galactose, maltose, fructose can be found in the ingredients lists on breakfast cereals labels and other processed and packaged products.

Starches: Americans consume most of their starches in the form of flour, rice, pasta, breads, cereals. Starches like whole grains, dried beans, dried peas, and sweet potatoes, however, are less likely choices.

While our intake of calories is very high, our intake of nutrients is inadequate for vibrant health. That's why the addition of dried barley leaves to our diet is such a simple, easy, quick way to supply the missing nutrients at an affordable price!

SUGAR AND DISEASE

About 80 percent of the carbohydrates you eat should be from the starch group and only 20 percent from the simple sugars. Since starch is a complex carbohydrate, it takes a much longer time to digest than sugar. Also, only 2 calories per minute go into the bloodstream from starch digestion while 10 calories per minute are released by the digestion of sugar.

Our organs, tissues, nerves, and other body parts react violently to the "flood" received when we eat a high sugar-content food or a pure carbohydrate food. Our bodies were not designed by their Creator to handle such excessive amounts of simple sugars.

Most Americans are eating 80 percent of their carbohydrates in the form of sugar and 20 percent in the form of starch. Why? Because it is easy to overdo on sugar consumption while eating what you think is starch. A hamburger bun from McDonald's, for instance, might not taste sweet to you, but sugar is a major ingredient in many starch products.

Many doctors with some nutrition training would give assent to a whole list of diseases caused or aggravated by our high sugar intake. Clearly, that list would include obesity, arteriosclerosis, heart disease, cancer, diabetes, arthritis, kidney stones, dental problems, high blood pressure, hyperactivity, hypoglycemia, and many others.

WHAT TO EAT

We hear a lot about fiber these days. Cellulose (plant fiber) is also a carbohydrate. The body's ability to digest cellulose is very poor, but it gives bulk and helps with the elimination of waste from the intestinal tract.

A friend of mine who is a medical doctor said in a lecture that 90 percent of bowel cancer could be eliminated by eating 2-3 tablespoons of bran and drinking 6-8 glasses of water daily.

Foods high in cellulose are: bran, dried fruits, legumes, fruits with skins, seedy fruits, green leafy vegetables (kale, collards, mustard greens, turnip greens, kohlrabi, etc.) and coarse fiber vegetables such as celery.[4]

Dr. Dennis Burkett, a surgeon who spent many years in South Africa, notes that in societies where the diet is composed of 80 percent complex carbohydrates (meaning starches), the people are healthy, robust, and free of many of our medical problems. Many studies have proved that vegetarians are healthier.

The body has a great backup system for making fantastic chemical adjustments quickly when we do foolish things such as drinking a quart of freshly squeezed orange juice (alkaline) at one sitting or eating a 16-oz. steak (acid) with lots of french fries (acid) and soda pop (acid) for dinner. Instead of depending on antacid tablets, we need to be more careful in planning our meals.[5]

You may find it interesting to compare qualities of certain foods in their ability to leave an acid or base residue in the body.

It is best to eat freely of the base-forming foods like: spinach, cucumbers, celery, lettuce, figs, fresh tomatoes, carrots, olives, parsnips, cabbage, cauliflower, fresh pineapple, orange juice, lemons, apricots, potatoes, raisins, squash, buttermilk, apples, pears.

Eat sparingly of acid-forming foods like: oysters, haddock, smelt, chicken, beef, eggs, halibut, mackerel, salmon, lamb, grains.

CAUSES OF ACIDOSIS

Many more people suffer from acidosis than alkalosis, and diet is only one factor involved here. Other than food intake, what causes acidosis? These are the most common:

Diarrhea. Among children, this is one of the most common causes of death.

Diabetes Mellitus. When a person cannot properly metabolize glucose, a rapid rise in acid production results.

Kidney Disease. Malfunctioning kidneys result in the third major cause of acidosis.

Vomiting. This may cause a loss of both acid and alkali and result in metabolic acidosis.

Stress. Mental, physical, emotional, and financial stress all produce an acid overload. There is no doubt that worry, fear, anxiety, jealousy, hatred, bitterness, anger, unforgiveness, and phobias of all kinds play havoc with the acid-base balance and our state of health.

Acidosis can also be caused by liver problems, shock, excess intake of salt, meat, fatty foods, obesity, fever, a too-rapid heartbeat, malnutrition, and many other things.

Remember, however, there are no medications available that can be dispensed to deal with the acids that are produced by negative thoughts, attitudes, and emotions. These things require spiritual, not physical, healing.

SYMPTOMS OF ACID STOMACH

What are the effects of acidosis?

Depression of the central nervous system. People first become depressed, then disoriented, and later can go into a coma, if they are not properly treated.

Heartburn. This is the most common symptoms of an imbalanced pH. A burning sensation in the pit of the stomach and burping of a highly acid liquid are sure symptoms of acidosis. Along with these, complaints of bloating, belching and a "full feeling" after a small amount of food are commonly reported.

There are a number of other symptoms one can observe that also indicate the presence of an acid excess. Here is a partial list: breathlessness, frequent sighing, irregular breathing, "cold sweat" perspiration, dryness of skin or mouth or throat, insomnia, hyperirritability, diminished urination, dry-hard stool, tachycardia (fast heartbeat), intolerance of light, restlessness, canker sores, easily broken or weak and peeling fingernails.[7]

If you have any of these symptoms, check with your doctor. "Acid indigestion," "sour stomach," and "heartburn" are signs that the body is having problems. Don't mistake heartburn for heart attack.

ANTACIDS — GOOD OR BAD?

What treatment should you consider if you have an acid stomach? Should you take products that contain sodium bicarbonate and other alkalinizing salts? Continued use of these easily-available, over-the-counter antacids may induce alkalosis, which causes your problems to become even more complex.

Before you begin to self-diagnose and self-medicate, however, I want you to hear an additional fact. Too little acid is also a common problem among the general population. According to one doctor who uses pH titration for measuring stomach acidity (few doctors test for this, actually), 35-50 percent of those tested had too little stomach acid rather than too much. This is especially true in patients who have been taking antacids regularly. In that group, more than 50 percent had below normal levels of acidity.

For years Americans have been bombarded on TV with clever ads leaving the impression that almost everyone needs an aid for faulty digestion. They come in liquid, tablet, capsule, and fizzing powder — all for the single purpose of neutralizing stomach acid.

Taking these products, however, does not in any way deal with the cause of too much acid, if indeed one exists. It simply masks the symptoms and makes your overall health worse if you are a habitual user over a long period of time.

If you are already a regular user of antacid products, on what basis did you make your choice of brand to be used? The ads we see on TV are not a scientifically sound basis for choosing between the more than 100 products available. Why? Because they tell the facts about tests in vitro (in a glass container), not in vivo (within the human body). Only what happens inside of us really matters!

ANTACID SIDE EFFECTS

If you are an antacid user, do you know the major ingredient of your antacid? Is there more than one active ingredient? Do you realize the dangers of masking symptoms which warn of the presence of serious illness?

Let's look at the most common antacids:

Sodium Bicarbonate. This is really ordinary baking soda, but it is extremely effective in neutralizing stomach acid, and it does its job rapidly. Problems, however, do exist with its use. Because of its efficiency in neutralizing acid, sodium bicarbonate can seriously upset the acid-base balance in the body, causing alkalosis.

It also contains very high amounts of sodium that anyone on a sodium-restricted diet or suffering from heart disease, kidney disease, or high blood pressure should avoid. People with poor kidney function need to stay away from it because it can lead to recurrent urinary tract infections (from urine becoming alkaline) and kidney stone formation with prolonged use.

In addition, several products, whose main ingredient is sodium bicarbonate, contain other ingredients, such as aspirin, which are actually harmful to an already irritated stomach lining! Be sure to check your labels before buying and taking these products.[8]

Magnesium. Available in one of several compounds, these are generally safe (except for those with chronic disease), but they have a laxative effect many people cannot tolerate.[9]

Aluminum Hydroxide. Although its action is good over a prolonged time, it is slow to begin to work and can cause severe constipation. Until recently, researchers believed that the body eliminated the aluminum present in medications. New findings indicate that some of it is absorbed into the bloodstream, and from there it can accumulate in other target areas, most notably the brain.[10]

This news is alarming, especially in light of the fact that the accumulation of aluminum in brain cells has been associated with Alzheimer's disease. Many of the best-selling antacids combine aluminum and magnesium compounds, causing the American's average daily consumption of aluminum to rise from 20 mgs. to 100 mgs. or more. Is the aluminum "load" from antacids poisoning us?

Calcium Carbonate. Probably the most effective antacid, it has no effect on the acid-base balance. It often causes constipation, however, requiring laxatives. It is another principal antacid found in numerous over-the-counter products. It, like sodium bicarbonate, works fast and is quite effective.

With prolonged or excessive use, calcium carbonate is capable of causing kidney malfunction and stone formation, as well as high blood calcium levels. If that's not bad enough, one study published in a prestigious medical journal reported that ingestion of calcium carbonate creates an "acid rebound" effect — that is, after temporarily neutralizing excess acid, it causes the body to produce even more acid as a result![11]

TV ads promote antacids as an effective source of calcium. Don't most Americans need more calcium? We have epidemic proportions of osteoporosis, weak backs, loose teeth, brittle fingernails, and many other conditions related to insufficient calcium supplies. What the ads don't tell us is that the calcium in antacids is nonusable for the most part because it does not contain the nutrients required for synergistic action with the calcium.

Barley leaves, not antacids, are an almost ideal product for this purpose. They are a rich natural source of calcium and have generous amounts of all the minerals required for its use.

SYMPTOMS OF ALKALOSIS

What are the symptoms, causes, and treatments for alkalosis?

The symptoms, actually, are often similar to those for acidosis. Determining which you have is sometimes difficult and requires the help of a professional.

Some common symptoms of excess alkali are: chronic indigestion, tiredness after eating a meal, heavy and slow pulse, night cramps, stiffness in joints, "thick" blood, high cholesterol, stone formation, osteoarthritis, asthma, "crawling sensation" of the skin, night coughs.[12]

As with acidosis, there are many possible causes of alkalosis. Some common ones are: diarrhea, vomiting, excess carbohydrate intake, stress, kidney disease, bronchitis, inflamed prostate, menopausal disorders, general endocrine imbalance, and others.

CHECKING YOUR OWN pH BALANCE

Two methods recommended for determining if your indigestion is due to an acid or alkaline imbalance are as follows:

• Drink four sips of an apple cider or wine vinegar mixture made from the following recipe: 2 tablespoons of vinegar in 1 cup of cool water. If you receive relief, you have alkalosis; if your heartburn is aggravated, you have acidosis.

• Place pH paper or litmus paper in the saliva of the mouth. Red litmus turns blue in an alkali media. Blue litmus turns red in an acid media.[13]

A pH BALANCED DIET

Balancing the diet with acid foods, taking extra vitamin C (which is acid) and a digestive pill containing hydrochloric acid will relieve alkalosis.

Alkali-forming minerals are sodium, potassium, calcium, and magnesium. Foods containing these minerals would be helpful in restoring a pH balance.

The typical American diet tends to produce "acid stomachs." Why? Because we are eating excessive amounts of foods such as meats, fish, poultry, sugar, soda pop, eggs, cheese, legumes, and cereals that burn and leave an acid ash. We eat much smaller amounts of alkaline-forming foods, which include vegetables, fruits, (except plums, prunes, rhubarb and cranberries) milk, and most nuts.

Dried barley juice is an excellent source of alkalinity to counter our acid-ash diet. This makes it truly a food with real power.

CHAPTER VIII

Keeping Your Battery Charged!

Barley leaves contain hundreds of "live" enzymes. Several of these have been isolated and studied for their healing properties.

What are enzymes? They are chemical substances required by every living cell for every biochemical process.

In breathing, for example, enzymes are involved in the exchange of oxygen and carbon dioxide in the lungs. They determine our responses to temperature changes. They are needed for reactions like muscle contraction, nerve conduction, urine excretion, and for almost everything else.

Enzymes actually fix not only the length of our lifespan but how effectively we maintain a high state of health and freedom from disease.

ENZYMES FOR A LIFETIME

If we lack enzymes needed for digestion, it might take us years to digest our supper. Every enzyme has a "life force" — a vitality at its very core — that is the body's labor force in maintaining health and healing. Scientists know there is a life principle, but they cannot assemble it in a test tube to be measured or studied.

Students of enzymology say that were it not for this life principle, humans would be no more than a heap of lifeless materials, a pile of dirt. Chemical substances of which we are made

— proteins, vitamins, minerals, and water — are lifeless and useless, they say, until acted upon in metabolism by the enzymes.[1]

This new theory also states that every person has a given, limited amount of enzyme energy at birth; it must last for the person's lifetime.

Enzymes are protein carriers charged with vital energy factors. Like the battery in your flashlight, the energy is exhaustible, and we must learn to conserve it.

DEPLETED ENZYMES LINKED TO ILLNESS

According to this theory, when we use up our enzyme supply quickly, such as by eating all cooked or processed foods that have no enzymes, our lives are shortened.[2] In addition to destroying enzymes by cooking, we also increase the need for them by eating "junk foods," drinking alcohol, smoking cigarettes, taking drugs, eating pork, shrimp, lobster, clams, catfish, etc., and by breathing impure air and drinking impure water, to name a few.

Depleting our enzyme supply results in a weakened immune system. Weakening our immune system results in making us prime targets for cancer, heart disease, arthritis, diabetes, obesity, AIDS, allergies, and many other degenerative diseases. As several researchers have pointed out, millions of North Americans experience death at middle-age instead of living out their full allotment of 70 years.

Why does this happen? Heavy withdrawals of enzymes are needed to digest an almost all-cooked diet, leading to eventual bankruptcy of the body's enzymes. As a result, the glands and the major organs, including the brain, suffer most.[3]

How can we prevent depleting our enzyme bank? By eating more raw foods such foods as raw milk, bananas, avocados, seeds, nuts, grapes, and other natural foods that are moderately high both in calories and food enzymes.

The digestion of a raw-food meal takes more time, but does not use up as many of the endogenous (made inside the body) digestive enzyme secretions (pancreatic juice, pepsin, erypsin, amylase, ptyalin, etc.) as does digestion of a cooked-food meal. This relieves the digestive burden of the organs and glands. It is also a way of sparing the life principle in enzymes so that, theoretically at least, the person lives longer, has better health, and has more enzyme potential for healing.[4]

ENZYMES AND WEIGHT CONTROL

Dr. Edward Howell believes that certain foods stimulate the pituitary gland (which is the body's secretion control center) and the pancreas (which secretes digestive enzymes for all three major types of food: protein, fat, and carbohydrates). Research shows that cooked foods excite these glands and tend to be fattening, while raw foods tend to be relatively nonstimulating and result in stabilized weight.[5]

This principle was shown in an experiment where the goal was to fatten hogs for market quickly and economically. Feeding hogs cooked potatoes produced the desired results even after the heavy cost of labor, etc., for the cooking of the potatoes.[6]

A study which confirmed these results was done on humans who were fed lots of fresh fruits (i.e., bananas, avocados, apples, oranges, etc.) and milk. The calorie intake was rather high, but the participants did not gain weight. The conclusion: cooked foods result in the production of more fat.[7]

Enzymes also seem to affect weight in other circumstances. Studies done in Germany and at the University of Illinois show rats had lower body weight and higher enzyme activity in the pancreas and fat cells when they ate only once a day.[8]

People who eat only one or two meals per day never seem to have a weight problem. A few, in fact, seem to be below the ideal weight for their age, sex, body build, and occupation but have a great deal of energy for sustained labor. These persons are, incidentally, adhering primarily to a vegetarian diet, which could be assumed to be higher in exogenous (made outside the body) enzymes.

CONSERVING THE ENZYME SUPPLY

When autopsies are performed, enzyme content of the pancreas widely differs. Those who died from cancer, diabetes, liver problems, and other debilitating diseases have markedly fewer enzymes in their pancreas than persons who were healthy when they died.[9]

Sick cells, especially cancer cells, rob the body of nutrients and prevent the production of enzymes. Thus, cancer cadavers, upon analysis, show a reduced enzyme level in their bodies.

How can we help conserve our enzyme supply? We must learn to eat daily a good supply of raw foods. All raw foods contain enzymes. No cooked foods have any enzymes left in them — none at all!

Blanching (scalding) bite-size pieces of green beans for more than one minute results in total enzyme loss. Heat destruction of enzymes begins at 107°F. and is complete at 122°F. So, no enzyme survives boiling (212°F.), and even enzymes in milk pasteurized at 145°F. are destroyed. That is why we must eat raw foods.

GOOD FOODS MADE BAD

The North American diet with its man-made, high-tech, "dead" foods has created a critical shortage of enzymes. Most, if not all, boxed products have been subjected to a number of processes involving high temperatures until they are enzymeless? So, the more your breakfasts and other meals are made of pre-prepared foods (in boxes, cans, or frozen), the more deficient you are in exogenous enzymes.

Chemists have identified 35 separate enzymes in raw milk, with lipase (the fat digesting enzyme) one of the chief factors. Undoubtedly, the high incidence of clogged arteries of North Americans is partly due to our high intake of homogenized milk — pasteurized milk with too few enzymes to make it digestible.[10] This nearly perfect food has been made harmful to consumers by completely changing milks chemical nature. More than 90 percent of the enzymes in milk are destroyed by modern-day pasteurization methods.

Unpasteurized milk and butter were used for thousands of years without conferring degenerative disease on their users. Why was that? Because the milk and butter were raw, and anything nature made for man's consumption as food contains the proper chemical substances to make it life-giving to the body. People lived for thousands of years without any atherosclerosis, heart disease, obesity, and other degenerative diseases that we suffer now in epidemic proportions.

When oil is converted into margarine, a good food becomes bad. Oils, in their natural state, are unsaturated fats that our bodies were designed to digest perfectly. The addition of hydrogen to those oils to make them into margarine and shortening creates a plastic-like material that the body has no digestive pathway for handling. All it can do is lay this material down in the arteries, thus creating circulation problems, hardening of the arteries, and eventual heart disease.

One physician said he believes margarine is the single most dangerous food on the American market!

Man has tampered with nature's perfect foods and turned them into a moneymaking operation that ignores the ill effects such processing has on the consumer. We are dying like flies from what the agri-business and commercial food giants have done to the food supply.

EATING GARBAGE CANS?

Another important way we can conserve our inherited supply of enzymes would be to follow the rules God gave the Israelites as recorded in the Bible. You can find these sensible dietary laws in the Old Testament books of Leviticus (chapter 11) and Deuteronomy (chapter 14).

One of the most outstanding examples is the command, "Eat no pig" (TLB). You don't need to be reminded that pork in its many forms (bacon, ham, sausage, ribs) is an all-American favorite. We love the taste of smoked, cured pork, and we eat it in very large quantities.

One doctor made the statement that because the pig is the "earth's garbage can," the consumption of pork requires thousands of enzymes to detoxify the flesh before the stomach can digest it. In the stomach and small intestine, it requires additional hundreds of enzymes to digest and assimilate it.

Because North Americans are short on enzymes, this doctor said that we are not adequately digesting the pork. It lies in our intestines, putrefies, forms carcinogens, and we show up with cancer. His advice was for us not to eat pork at all.

Do you want to live a long, healthy, disease-free life? Then, as much as possible, eliminate pork from your diet. You should also eliminate shrimp, catfish, lobster, oysters, and clams from your diet. Why? Because they are the "garbage cans" of the rivers and oceans. Consuming them is extremely destructive to the limited supply of our enzymes.

If we will make these sacrifices of eating pleasure, we will live longer, healthier, and more productive lives, while we greatly reduce our risk of dying from some of our worst killer diseases.

ENZYMES: KEY TO LONGEVITY?

As we grow older, there seems to be diminished secretion of enzymes in the stomach and intestinal tract. This results in poor digestion and assimilation and a malnourished condition that results in a weakened body with less vitality. Death overtakes those with depleted enzymes more quickly than those whose enzymes remain strong enough to digest and assimilate their food.

Cancer centers in other countries are successfully using enzymology as a treatment modality for this killer disease. Perhaps this is one of the reasons why their cure rate is so superior to the American standard procedure! An international study has now proven that chemotherapy, radiation, drugs, and surgery are not the answers to cancer! It is reported that Dr. Hans Nieper of Hanover, West Germany, has a 74 percent cancer cure rate compared to 17 percent in the United States.

In his treatment of cancer patients, Dr. Nieper uses enzyme therapy in addition to a strict vegetarian diet. He uses almost no drugs and absolutely no chemotherapy or radiation. Wouldn't it be wonderful if American doctors would at least give us a choice in treatment modalities for degenerative diseases? This is true especially regarding the "Big Four" — heart disease, cancer, diabetes, and atherosclerosis.

VITAMIN HELPERS

Can you see, now, why we must eat fresh, raw foods every day? Is your food intake "live" or "dead" when it comes to enzymes. Remember, no enzymes, no digestion; no enzymes, no assimilation; no digestion or assimilation, no vibrant health — and certainly no resistance to killer diseases.

Raw fruits and vegetables are essential to a healthy diet. Dried barley juice is a raw food, and it contains hundreds of "live" enzymes.

Digestive enzymes do not work alone, however, they have quite a host of helpers called co-enzymes. Vitamins are in this category. That being true, it is also easy to see the importance of getting enough (but not too much) of the vitamins required for optimal enzymatic function.

Do we need to supplement our diet with vitamin pills? It will be wonderful when scientists can accurately assess the status of the body's vitamin levels. Until then, I believe modest supplementation is a good idea.

From our chemically treated soil, to our chemically processed foods, packed in chemically treated packages, who knows what the vitamin and mineral content of today's foods actually is?

When a new crop of cabbage was tested for its vitamin C value, the farmer was shocked to find that the amount of vitamin C in his sample was too small to register on the equipment being used by the government agency. Unfortunately, this is not an isolated case.

Carrots grown by a Pennsylvania farmer for years had always measured around 16 on a refractometer to gauge the carrots' mineral level, using a scale from 1 to 22. In recent years, as modern farming methods replaced organic farming, his carrots have measured only four to six!

Unfortunately, we consumers are the ones who are registering, if not suffering, the loss. The farmer's profit on his crops has probably remained fairly constant, if not increased a bit.

YOU ARE WHAT YOU DIGEST

Nature has placed within each food on this planet — both plant and animal — specific enzymes needed for at least the beginning stages of its digestion.

Enzymes are not only found in raw, unprocessed food, but two types are also produced inside the body. These digestive enzymes are synthesized by the glands and organs of the digestive tract.

Another enzyme category is metabolic enzymes — products of the endocrine glands (thyroid, parathyroid, adrenal, and pituitary). These enzymes build, repair, and maintain the functioning of every organ, tissue, and cell. They actually build the body from proteins, carbohydrates and fats. Without them, life is impossible.

In fact, old age and worn-out metabolic enzyme activity are always twin concepts. You don't see one without the other. This is also true in the lives of mammals other than man.

Following digestion in the mouth, in the stomach, and in the small intestine, food must be assimilated (absorbed by our 78 to 83 trillion cells) before it gives life to the body. Thus, we are not what we eat as much as we are what we digest and metabolize because of the quantity and quality of enzymes in our system.

STRESS AT THE SALAD BAR

The typical American diet is overheated, overcooked, and overprocessed, which makes it enzyme-deficient. This means the pancreas, salivary glands, and other organs are unable to carry through on their natural responsibilities. As a result, we experience belching, burning in the stomach, gas in the intestines and many other unpleasantly familiar symptoms.

Good enzymic action is necessary for life, and it is not possible to have good enzyme action when the necessary nutrients are lacking in your body. These nutrients will not be present for your use unless you eat a proper diet or take adequate supplements on a regular basis.

Research shows that eating simple meals instead of complex ones affects enzyme requirements. Meals containing many different kinds of food are difficult to digest. Why? Because each food requires its very own set of enzymes.

A typical American salad bar meal, containing small amounts of many foods is a stressful situation for the body. This is especially true when we complicate the problem by adding large quantities of salad dressing.

High-calorie intake is also related to degenerative diseases such as obesity, heart disease, and especially cancer.

BURSTING WITH "LIVE" ENZYMES

The green leaves of the embryonic barley plant are an excellent source of hundreds of "live" enzymes. This statement cannot be made for any man-made vitamin or mineral tablet. Most lack natural enzymes and, probably, enzymes from any source.

Barley leaves, in the raw state, are an excellent source of enzymes and co-enzymes (vitamins) required for the body's biochemical reactions. It is easy for me to believe they create the best possible atmosphere for healthy cell activity to flourish.

Research has also produced evidence that suggests enzyme supplements should be used just as regularly and as faithfully as vitamin and mineral supplements. This is particularly true when people are older or suffering from a disease robbing them of the life-force needed to create enzymes. Enzyme supplements should also be taken if we are not including generous quantities of raw foods in our daily food intake.

If you are having difficulty with digestion and decide you might like to try enzyme supplementation, there are a number of good products available at drugstores or health-food stores. When taken before meals, they work more or less like those digestive enzymes made by the body.

One single food has a worldwide reputation for dynamic enzymatic power — the embryonic leaves of the barley plant. Barley leaves are the ideal, instant-food way for busy Americans to get their daily serving of raw, leafy greens.

CHAPTER IX

Living Longer and Better

According to Dr. Hagiwara, the juice from the young barley plants may contain thousands of enzymes; about 300 already have been isolated. These enzymes correspond to those found in the human body cells. It is this multitude of enzymes, saved intact and "alive" by his method for making dried barley juice that sets it absolutely in a class by itself.

"ON GUARD" AGAINST TOXINS

Enzymes neutralize poisons in the body. Specific enzymes in dried barley juice can help purge the body of toxins that we absorb as pollutants in the air, water, and food we consume.

Almost all chemical substances and environmental pollutants have carcinogenicity — the ability to produce cancers of many types. Seventy percent of carcinogens are nitric compounds, which are petroleum solvents.

Barley juice contains nitrate reductase, which has been proven to act as an antidote to these poisonous nitro-compounds. Barley juice is also particularly rich in two additional enzymes that can help nutritionally strengthen the body to resist and counteract mutations.

Dr. Hagiwara and his research staff have isolated one barley juice molecule, which they have named P_4D_1. It definitely lessens the cancer-producing ability of the typical nitro-oxides and can also counteract toxic effects of BHT— a chemical used to preserve many food products.[1]

Of special importance is the fact that this peroxidase is more active in an acidic environment. Therefore, one would expect that barley leaves may possibly even begin decomposing cancer-producing substances in the stomach, where the digestive juices are highly acidic.[2]

Also, P_4D_1 has been found to have an anti-peptic ulcer and anti-inflammatory function but with no side effects as with ordinary anti-inflammatory drugs. It is thought to be superior to cortisone and non-steroid drugs (which have a common side effect of producing ulcers), such as phenylbutazone, widely used today as treatment for these problems.[3]

Many chemicals, including artificial food additives, can distort the human design genetically, resulting in birth defects. It is also clear DNA breakage is involved in the development of some cancers.

Barley juice definitely contains elements which, by decomposing and dissolving certain mutagens, can reduce the risk of your having to share space with tobacco smokers and can help prevent cancer and counteract mutations in already damaged DNA.

If you work around exhaust fumes, industrial chemicals, dry-cleaning fluids, pesticides, or other substances of these sorts, the best thing you can do for yourself is to take a teaspoon or two of dried barley juice a day.

LOOK BETTER LONGER

The juice from green barley leaves is definitely one of the best general detoxifiers. It's full of flavonoids, which detoxify the cellular tissue, as well as polypeptides, which can neutralize nicotine and heavy metals, like mercury, into insoluble salts. Everything about it helps to strengthen the organs that purge the bloodstream and excrete the toxins.

Damage to the DNA/genes occurs from various other factors as well: ultraviolet light, cosmic rays, and radiation, for example. Most of these damages can be repaired by natural defense systems, but some get misrepaired while others can accumulate in the genome (a set of chromosomes) due to a weak repair system.[4]

The stronger and more accurate the repair activity in our cells, the better it is for our health and ability to maintain youthful characteristics. Our repair activity gets weaker as we get older, and the damage keeps accumulating. Damage to cellular DNA can relate to the introduction of cancer, allergy, or the death of cells in our body.[5]

Researchers have found that green barley juice powder promotes the restoration of damaged DNA in the cell's nucleus.[6] Barley juice has the potential to help protect us from ever-increasing environmental hazards and forced aging, and perhaps even to postpone the natural aging process itself.

CATALASE AND CANCER

Green barley juice contains another enzyme that researchers are looking into as a potential therapy — the respiratory enzyme catalase.

An experimental report suggests that milk may reduce catalase activity in the body fluids. This would lead to a rise in hydrogen peroxide in the course of metabolism, adversely affecting the cells. Another experimental report showed that a milk-containing meal also decreased the level of cytochrome oxidase, which is also an important respiratory enzyme.[7]

These enzymes cannot be formed unless there are plenty of iron and copper ions in the blood. Milk, however, has a low content of copper and iron, as do other staples of the North American diet: butter, polished rice, and bleached bread. Too much of these foods can weaken the activities of these important enzymes in our body, resulting in cancer.

SUPER ENZYMES

Researchers around the world are busy investigating a host of recently discovered practical applications for super-oxide dismutase (SOD). (A potent SOD tablet is available under the name "Superzymes" from the distributors of BarleyGreen).

SOD's chief function, in contrast to other enzymes, is as a cell protector. It ferrets out and destroys the hazardous active forms of oxygen that are constantly being produced as chemical by-products of cellular metabolism in the course of respiration and digestion.

Superoxides, or free radicals, are the "bad guys." Natural nutrients, including superoxide dismutase, which destroy them are the "good guys." It is important to have a good supply of SOD in our bodies, especially if we are ill with one of the diseases related to a free radical problem, like heart problems, arthritis, cancer, leukemia, allergies, and lupus.

SOD has been shown to:
- Reduce the inflammation of arthritis.
- Aid in the healing of wounds.
- Greatly aid damaged heart, kidney, intestines, pancreas, and skin tissue.
- Reduce the number and severity of abnormal heart rhythms, called arrythmias.
- Act as a cell protector — a main function.
- Reduce chances of getting cancer and a host of other degenerative diseases.
- Slow down the aging process.
- Alleviate symptoms related to radiation sickness.[8]

After a heart attack, cellular energy production is severely lowered. Prevention or delay of irreversible cell damage can be achieved by simply administering enzymes specifically aimed at maintaining the energy supply of the cell. SOD is one of these enzymes that increases the efficiency of energy production.

Dried barley juice is an excellent natural source of SOD.

DIGESTIVE ENZYME SUPPLEMENTATION

Research suggests that enzyme supplements are as important to good health as vitamin and mineral supplements. Of course, you know which enzyme supplement I believe is the best — the powdered juice of young barley leaves! But for those with special needs for digestive enzymes, I can make the following suggestions.

Digestive enzyme supplementation is especially important to those who:

- Do not include generous quantities of leafy green and yellow vegetables and other raw foods in the daily diet.
- Are elderly and/or under continuous stress.
- Have difficulty with digestion.
- Are suffering from any of the degenerative diseases (heart disease, hypertension, cancer, diabetes, etc.).

There are a number of good products available. Taken according to directions, they work much like digestive enzymes made by the body. In shopping for a digestive enzyme supplement, read labels carefully. Unless you know your exact needs from clinical testing, it seems logical to buy a broad spectrum product that aids in digesting proteins, fats and carbohydrates (phone us for a recommendation).

Full-spectrum digestive-aid tablets often contain enzymes that work in the stomach or the duodenum. Once opened, these products should be kept in a dark, cool, dry place!

REVERSING THE AGING PROCESS?

Research studies show that SOD protects the cells from free radical damage. Since it is known that free radicals damage cells and damaged cells begin to die, contributing to aging, could it be that the SOD could reverse the aging process? Many studies have concluded that it can and it does.

Aging begins in cells and tissues that are denied the nutritional support they need for reproduction, for repairing the damage done daily by toxins, by poisons, dyes, chemicals, carcinogens, radiation, illness, lack of enzymes, and the lack of oxygen and water. Dried green barley juice is nutritional therapy for so many of these cell problems. Its excellent balance of vitamins B_1, B_2, B_6, B_{12}, nicotinic acid, vitamins A, E and C, as well as a wide spectrum of minerals, certainly offers a nutritional impact on cell and tissue health while protecting the body against aging and a shortened life span.

While it may prove true that SOD can delay the aging process somewhat, science will never find an ultimate cure for either aging or death. We die because a mortogenic factor was introduced into our race by a man named Adam, and SOD can't change that fact. However, there is every indication that SOD can provide a better chance of a decent quality of life into advanced old age.

REPAIRING DAMAGED CELLS

Studies support the value of green barley juice in giving support to cells that have been damaged by radiation. All forms of radiation produce free radicals, including excessive exposure to the sun, to computer and TV screens, X-rays, food irradiation, microwave ovens, and fall-out from atomic waste. Research also shows that SOD can inhibit tumor promotion.[9]

Clearly, sources in our enzyme family, especially SOD, glutathione peroxidase, methione reductase, and catalase, are the most powerful antioxidants our body uses as a first line of defense to fight radiation free radicals. Fortunately for us, nature has a cure. The answer lies in the quality and quantity of our nutrient intake from all sources, including enzyme supplementation.

Nature has provided us with a food — barley leaves — which has the power, through enzymes and co-enzymes (in addition to amino acids, minerals, chlorophyll, etc.), to provide our cells with the basic weapons needed for both health and fighting disease. The decision to incorporate a teaspoon or two of dried barley juice into your daily diet would be one of the best (and most economical) ways to assure yourself of an improved quality of life.

Barley leaves are truly food with real enzymatic power!

CHAPTER X

Daily Nutrient Power

Research shows that daily eating carrots and green vegetables can help your body fight cancer. Scientists conclude that beta-carotene protects phagocytic cells from free radical damage. It increases the production of T and B lymphocytes and enhances the ability of macrophage, cycotoxic cells, and natural killer cells to reverse tumor and cancer cell growth.[1] And without any damaging side-effects.

If you eat too much beta-carotene, which is practically impossible, there is a recipe in the cell for getting rid of the excess without any cell, tissue, or organ damage. That's more than we can say for synthetic drugs.

Research done with rats showed that infections of the ear, bladder, kidney, and gut were prevented and/or reversed when adequate amounts of beta-carotene were included in the diet. Young children with chronic ear infections always showed improvement with increased intake of dietary carotene.[2] Why then do most M.D.'s use antibiotics (with their high cost, high health risk, and low cure rate) instead of beta-carotene?

How much beta-carotene do you need every day? Authorities differ in their answers. A study showed that a single 30 milligram capsule of beta-carotene (equivalent to the amount in about six carrots) reversed premalignant leukoplakia in more than 75 percent of the patients without producing any toxic side effects.[3]

Most authorities agree that a *daily* serving of one-half cup of a deep-green leafy vegetable (collards, turnip greens, kale, spinach) or a serving of a deep-yellow vegetable (sweet potatoes, squash, carrots) is considered adequate for good health.

Since powdered barley leaves have generous amounts of beta-carotene, it is one more reason to take one to two teaspoons daily. That would certainly go a long way toward meeting our beta–carotene need in an inexpensive "instant food" way.

TOO MUCH OF A GOOD THING

We need sufficient amounts of all the vitamins. Foods naturally high in vitamins do little good, however, when consumed in processed form. Why? Because vitamins can be altered during processing.

For example, the iron component will change under heat to iron oxide, which is not easily absorbed by the body. To treat anemia, iron preparations containing iron reduced to this form are popular but not very serviceable for blood formation. Since green barley contains iron in the organically bonded state (divalent iron), it can be immediately absorbed from the intestinal tract.

The vitamins in green barley have not been isolated and then recombined, but are still in their natural (chelated) form, bonded to other nutrient factors as nature created them. If you throw together similar amounts of isolated or man-made chemicals, you will not produce the same effect.

Many health enthusiasts have gone "vitamin crazy." While synthetic vitamins provide many immediate beneficial results, vitamins — especially isolated vitamins — can throw off the body's balance.

Hyper-vitaminosis, caused by excessive vitamin ingestion, is almost always associated with synthetic vitamin preparations — but hardly ever with natural vitamins. Since green barley contains vitamins in their natural state, its use will not result in an excessive intake of any particular vitamin.

For example, excess vitamin A can be harmful — but only when it is pure vitamin A taken in high quantities. Carotene in green barley is called provitamin A, and it becomes vitamin A only as acted upon by the body. It cannot cause hyper-vitaminosis.

THE SAFEST AND SUREST SOURCE

Green barley is an excellent source of live, natural vitamins and, I believe, is sufficient as the only food supplement. But if you are accustomed to taking more vitamins than in green barley, you might want to continue your regular dosage right along with the green barley.

Personally, I take two multivitamins and also 1 to 3 teaspoons of green barley a day and feel better than I did with the multivitamins alone.

Whichever way you go, I recommend taking only vitamins extracted from food, not synthetic ones. Although in the laboratory many synthetic vitamins appear to be no different from those extracted from nature, I wonder if they react differently in the body than they do in the test tube.

The safest and surest source of good nutrition comes from grains, legumes, vegetables (including green plants), and fruits. Adverse effects inevitably follow ingestion of large quantities of unnatural food of unbalanced organic-inorganic nature. Five grams of green barley juice contains as much Vitamin A as two bananas; nearly the same amount of Vitamin B_1 as an average serving of cabbage; more Vitamin B_2 than a serving of potatoes; twice as much Vitamin C as two apples.

MINERALS: ALL OF THEM

All living organisms are born and die with minerals as their axis. Man was made from clay. When either a plant or a human body is burned, the same minerals remain in the ashes. Unlike plants, however, the human body cannot draw necessary minerals directly out of its environment or manufacture them. Our only source for minerals is in food we eat.

Why do we need minerals? Among other functions, minerals maintain the pH balance in our bodies. When we lose our acid-alkaline balance, our cell metabolism suffers. This can lead to all sorts of trouble. Our cells maintain this balance by constantly absorbing, consuming, and discharging various minerals.

Enzymes, agents that make metabolism possible, work only if the right minerals are dissolved as ions in our cell fluids. All chemical changes within our cells require enzyme action, and minerals have so much to do with the action of enzymes that they may be called the enzymes for the enzymes!

When the right minerals are not present in an ionized condition, most enzymes cease functioning effectively, often completely. When foods with proper mineral content are neglected, or when foods with high concentrations of the wrong minerals are consumed heavily, the body cannot prosper.

WHERE HAVE ALL THE MINERALS GONE?

The American diet is short on minerals because it is short on vegetables and grains. The skeleton of a man who died today would yield less potassium and other minerals than the skeleton of a man who died at the turn of the century.

Not only do we eat fewer mineral-rich foods, but those we eat are of diminished mineral content. "Factory" farming methods, besides polluting the soil with industrial chemicals, bleach it chemically of its inherent energy. Also, nitrogen compounds are released into the air by automobiles and industry, where they change to nitric and sulfuric acid (acid rain).

This "acid rain" is progressively dissolving the alkaline metals in our soil, robbing it of potassium and magnesium and other minerals essential to the vitality of all forms of life. Most of the fruits and vegetables we buy today have been grown in such soil by such methods and are of diminished vitality from those of even 50 years ago.

SALT: NOT THE WAY IT USED TO BE

At the same time, we tend to be getting too much of certain minerals like phosphorus and, especially, sodium (salt). Two grams daily of salt is sufficient for human beings, but most of us consume 10 times that much.

Natural salt contains bittern with minerals like potassium, calcium, and magnesium that are absent in our modern product. The salt we use today, however, is made by ion exchange membrane methods and is a reagent-grade chemical, 99.9 percent pure sodium chloride. A fish will live for a week in a solution of natural salt but will die in a few hours in a solution made from what's in our salt shakers today.

Salt exerts great effects on our cells, and the mineral deficiency in our present species of table salt should be regarded as a serious matter. I believe it is linked to our loss of health in general, and, especially, to the increase in heart disease, hypertension, and fatigue.

Pay the extra pennies to put the natural sea salt on your table, and even then be careful not to eat too much salt.

WHY POTASSIUM IS IMPORTANT

Green barley is very high in potassium, which works to balance the sodium excess in our diets. Potassium has a very high ionizing tendency and is consumed incessantly within our bodies in the process of energy metabolism. When potassium levels fall too low, sodium increases above a healthy limit. As a result, the balance of ions within the cell fluid is disrupted. Some enzymes continue to work, but others falter or stop functioning altogether.

Modern diets tend to foster this condition because the proportion of acidic foods (such as meat, starch, and sugars) is large, and that of alkaline foods (primarily vegetables and fruits) is minor. Over-consumption of acidic foods — with only small amounts of potassium — is involved in a broad range of disease conditions.

Many have attributed high blood pressure, heart disease, and circulatory disease partially to over-consumption of salt and high sodium levels. Many drugs that alleviate high sodium levels also tend to deplete the body of potassium. The result may be lowered blood pressure or fatigue because of potassium lack. Research shows that, if potassium is simply added to the diet, it balances and neutralizes the sodium levels and helps to lower the blood pressure.

DANGER: LOW POTASSIUM

Hypokalemia results from a reduced potassium concentration in the blood. Symptoms include body languor (weakness), especially muscular fatigue, and can lead to paralysis. Furthermore, cirrhosis hepatitis is, in a sense, a disease associated with loss of potassium.

Many medicines lower our potassium level dangerously. When a diuretic or cortisone is administered, excretion of potassium from body fluids increases abruptly. Dr. Hagiwara says when such a therapy is practiced, potassium in a completely natural form should be supplied at the same time.[4]

The motion of muscles also involves a release of potassium. Our heart and blood vessels continue to contract and relax from birth to death without a moment's rest. What happens if potassium is not supplied sufficiently for the working of your heart and blood vessels? The muscles strongly resist releasing potassium, and if the potassium deficiency is exacerbated by continued consumption of acidic foods containing much fat but few minerals, cholesterol and wastes build up in the blood vessels.

Heart diseases of the middle and old-aged, such as myocardial infarction, mostly afflict those who eat luxuriously and seem to be exposed to much stress. Stress itself also involves a release of potassium. Potassium in green barley can help improve these conditions and serve to prevent heart disease.

FEELING TIRED?

How could all these diseases be related to something so simple as a lack of potassium? Your automobile might provide a good analogy. It's made to run with five quarts of oil. Insist on operating it with two quarts, and you'll eventually ruin everything from the water pump to the wiring (and lots of things in between). Our bodies are like that. Deny the whole body what it was meant to "run on" and it will eventually start breaking down all over.

The first sign of potassium shortage is usually fatigue. The fatigue that attends strenuous physical exertion and mental activity, or stress and the fatigue following lack of sleep differ metabolically, but they all share one common denominator — a build-up of sodium and loss of potassium. Too much salt or too little potassium will result in tension and muscular fatigue.

Dr. Hagiwara asks, "What happens to those who continuously follow a diet deficient in potassium?" Since the body has a self-defending system, there will be an effort to store potassium within the cells. If complete loss of potassium is threatened, the body tries to prevent secretion of potassium. Consequently, our bodies are forced to stop all strong muscular exercise.

"Exertions of the brain or nerves, which consume greater energy than physical labor, become dull. This in turn causes the body to stop releasing potassium and results in sleepiness and languidness. If you noticed this and took potassium, the cells would regain vigor and resume energy metabolism."[5]

If you are always tired, try green barley and see if it doesn't make a difference. I have eaten "right" for years, yet it gives me more energy — and I believe it will help you as well.

PHOSPHORUS BALANCER

The other mineral we get too much of is phosphorus, especially phosphoric acid. Experiments show that as the amount of phosphoric acid increases, so do occurrences of bone malformation. Increased phosphoric acid in the feed of pregnant mice produces a proportional increase of malformed fetuses.

Stay away from phosphoric acid, and, most especially, from fizzy soft drinks. They're refreshing for the moment, but they're trouble in the long run. Give them up and don't let your children drink them. They will ruin teeth and bones and upset other calcium functions.

For example, hypocalcemia is a disease resulting from the reduction of calcium concentration in blood. It manifests itself in bone troubles, osteomalacia, abnormal excitation of nerves, or a disordered condition of the parathyroid gland. I can't prove it, so I'd better not say what my suspicion is about the cause of Kaschin-Beck disease, but, please, most especially if you're pregnant, *avoid phosphoric acid!*

Many of the foods we eat, including meat, are high in phosphorus and low in calcium. Green barley is the reverse and can help balance out the surplus phosphorus, promoting better utilization of all minerals. A deficiency in any one mineral will upset our ability to profit from the others. (For example, both hypokalemia and hypocalcemia can be induced by the deficiency of a magnesium ion in body fluids.)

Dried barley juice has a wider range, higher quantity, and better balance of minerals than any of the foods that are commonly valued for mineral content. Because of the small percentage of kelp in it, green barley also has trace amounts of all the 14 other minerals, including molybdenum, iodine, germanium, selenium, and lithium, all in their raw organic forms. The minerals in green barley have not been freeze-dried and are still in their original easily absorbable biochemical form.

Five grams of green barley has more calcium than an average serving of cabbage or green beans; more phosphorus than a banana or an orange; more iron than a serving of broccoli or corn; more than twice as much potassium as a serving of brussels sprouts or potatoes or peaches.

What better way to supplement your diet and meet your nutritional needs?

CHAPTER XI

Food Power in Action

Our main purpose in writing this book on the dried juice of young barley leaves is to encourage North Americans, and people everywhere, to improve their declining health through improving their diet.

Believing as I do that the best, easiest, quickest, least expensive single way of improving the nutrient density of your diet is by the daily addition of a serving of green leaves of barley, I have done my best to introduce you to the scientific facts about it. Hopefully many of you will also want to read my books entitled, *Green Leaves of Barley, Nature's Miracle Rejuvenator* and *The Spiritual Roots of Barley.* These add a deep dimension to the subject of barley.

The next step is up to you. Making wise food choices and providing nutritious meals for yourself and family has a price tag attached. But remember this: *Neglecting* to get serious about your nutritional health has a much higher price.

More than a year of my life has been invested in writing these books. If as a result of reading them, you take the positive steps to improve your diet, write to me and share what you have done— what changes you have made. My address is: Dr. Mary Ruth Swope, P.O. Box 5075, Scottsdale, Arizona 85261.

DISCLAIMER
Unsolicited testimonies are included solely for the purpose of nutrition information and education. Nothing in this book should be construed as medical advice.

Products made from raw, young, green barley leaves in the form of barley juice powder have no medical properties. They are not, therefore, intended for the cure, mitigation, prevention, or treatment of any disease, illness, or symptom.

Please consult your physician or other qualified health professional should your health problems warrant the need for one.

[Note: Hereafter, this symbol [n.n] ("no name") is being used to represent the brand of green barley juice represented in the following testimonies.]

MY CUSTOMERS SPEAK

I will let the words of my customers speak for themselves. These testimonies are only a few of the many hundreds I have received over the years. The first two are from medical doctors who asked to remain anonymous.

RESISTING DEGENERATIVE DISEASE

In my medical practice I have recommended green barley to many of my patients, and most have reported significant improvement almost immediately. I have seen improvement in patients with arthritis, asthma, diabetes, lupus, tonsillitis, sinus problems, chronic and excessive fatigue, colitis, and other GI problems, and various skin problems, including roughness, brown spots, and acne.

Clearly, green barley boosts the immune system. It provides powerful support to the body's own health-promoting mechanisms, and I firmly believe it can help the body arm itself to resist the assaults of the "Big Four": diabetes, heart disease, hypertension, and cancer. It is the most effective general antidote for nutritional debilitation that I know of, bar none. Plus, it is safe, it tastes okay, and it is priced right.

BALANCING, CLEANSING, AND HEALING

I was very skeptical when first introduced to [n.n] in September, 1982. I tried it on myself and my family and a few select patients, and soon became impressed with a number of very good results in a wide variety of conditions. Just in the last five months, I have observed improvement in the following areas: allergies, asthma, emphysema, a variety of skin conditions, tendonitis, bursitis, arthritic pain, reduction of blood pressure, improved regularity and elimination, improvement in cases of gastritis, pancreatitis, peptic ulcers, diabetes, hypoglycemia, gum disease, lessening of symptoms in menopause and PMS, and decrease of toxic symptoms in chemotherapy.

Because [n.n] is a high-quality, balanced, natural green food product, it helps the body balance, cleanse, and heal itself.

CONGESTION, HAY FEVER, AND HIVES
For a long time, I had problems with hives and hay fever. I had a lot of nose and chest congestion accompanied by sneezing and coughing. After 2-1/2 months of taking [n.n] (two teaspoons a day), the hay fever is almost nonexistent. The hives only bother me when I have vinegar on a salad and then only a light case. What a difference!

—R28, Tallahassee, FL

RHEUMATOID ARTHRITIS AND ALLERGIES
I am finishing my first jar of [n.n], and my sinus problems, hay fever, and allergies are completely gone. I am noticing the swelling from my rheumatoid arthritis is getting less everyday since I started [n.n]. I believe it is a real Godsend and I'm looking forward to continued healing.

—L49, Los Angeles, CA

RHEUMATOID ARTHRITIS, HYPOGLYCEMIA
It was just after a very stressful time, when my arthritis had hit hard, that we found [n.n]. Since I've been taking it, the rheumatoid arthritis seems to be going into remission, and I have more energy than before. I have hypoglycemia, and with the [n.n] my blood sugar level stays level too. [n.n] gives me a steady stream of energy that carries me all day.

—R10, Monett, MO

NO MORE COUGHING

My 4-year-old son used to be up coughing almost every night, even with cough syrup. Since starting on [n.n], his coughing has stopped and his asthma is tremendously improved. We can sleep at night now, and are very grateful for that.

—L135, Bethany, OK

EMPHYSEMA AND BRONCHIAL ASTHMA

I have emphysema and bronchial asthma, so I have had a problem with recurring colds and pneumonia. Since taking [n.n], I just don't get sick as often. I feel it builds up the immune system.

—R3, Indialantic, FL

OAT CELL CANCER IN REMISSION

My husband was diagnosed as terminal four months ago, with oat cell carcinoma. He is to receive the fifth of six doses of chemotherapy next week. With the help of [n.n], he has tolerated the regime well. The doctor says that since he is gaining weight and his kidneys and bowels are functioning better than they ever have, plus his diabetes is under control, he considers the cancer in remission

—L23, Romulus, MI

CANCER OF THE LIVER

Good news — scans last week reveal shrinkage of the liver tumor. The specialist is very encouraged, as are we. Doubtless chemotherapy played an important part, but I'm convinced [n.n] also deserves credit. Before starting [n.n], there had been stabilization, but no shrinkage.

—L66, St. Louis, MO

CANCER OF THE COLON

I have been taking [n.n] for five months. Before I started, I had been operated on for cancer of the colon, and was feeling tired and run down. Since starting [n.n], I feel stronger, and my checkup showed no further cancer. The doctor says I am in good condition

—R72, Bangor, PA

LUMPS IN BREASTS RECEDE

Last Spring I noticed lumps in both breasts. They measured about 7 centimeters each. Then I started taking [n.n]. When I went in for a recheck in December, the doctor said they measured less than six centimeters each, and there was no need for a biopsy.

—T91, Melbourne, FL

HIGH CHOLESTEROL

After surviving two aneurysms in 1986, I am under medical monitoring every six weeks. I started on [n.n]. Between one appointment and the next, my blood levels of cholesterol and triglycerides showed a pronounced change for the better. Also, an added bonus: my breath is vastly more palatable. Besides, I seem to have a higher energy level.

—K75, San Diego, CA

HYPERTENSION, GOUT

We can tell we are improving by using [n.n]. It has made me feel more energetic, stopped my tendonitis, and improved my husband's blood pressure and gout. The doctor was very much surprised with my husband's progress. The symptoms [n.n] has cleared up, for my husband, were weakness, irritability, headaches, and depression. My stiff joints had pains like pins and needles. Another nice thing about [n.n]; it helps sore throats as well as sore joints!

—R27, Fyffe, AL

SORE THROATS, COLDS, AND ALLERGIES

Before [n.n], I had to watch constantly against sore throats and colds. I have had some difficulties with allergies as well. I started taking [n.n] last fall; now I hardly know what a sneeze is! This is the first winter I can say I have been without a cold.

—R58, Austin, TX

LOOSE TEETH, BLEEDING GUMS

Before I started taking [n.n], I had loose teeth and sore gums that would bleed at the slightest touch and when I brushed my teeth. Now I no longer have any sign of gum disease, plus I have been healed of several long-time ailments. I have had headaches all my life, but since taking [n.n], they're gone. It has helped my eyesight, and my muscle and joint problems are still improving. I feel great, have lots of energy, and am very alert and organized. Also, my husband's ulcer has been no problem since he's been taking it.

—R81, Vancouver, WA

INTESTINAL CLEANSING

After starting [n.n], I felt weak, and noticed a lot of bowel elimination was taking place. There was also pain throughout my body, as well as fatigue. This took four days of cleansing, and I rested as much as possible during that period. Since that time, I feel better and better everyday.

—L98

pH OF URINE

I am excited about the way [n.n] brought my acid urine pH up in no time at all and has kept it alkaline. I have been working to bring my system into a slightly alkaline pH range for four years now. No other food I have ever used was as effective as [n.n]. I spent a year at *The Saturday Evening Post* as a food editor, so I am familiar with the nutritional principles [n.n] puts to work in us.

—L96, Fortville, IN

BREAKING THE CAFFEINE HABIT

Since I started taking [n.n], I have stopped drinking coffee. I drink [n.n] in the morning to get going instead—it works great!

—R12, Uniontown, OH

BREAKING THE SUGAR HABIT

With [n.n] I have more energy and less craving for sweets. Within one week, my energy level improved so much I just didn't want sweets.   —R69, San Diego, CA

CONTROL OF BLOOD SUGAR LEVEL

My wife has had diabetes for five years. She started out on pills, then about five years ago had to go on shots. Just at the point where we were going to have to increase her insulin, she started on [n.n]. Now she will not need to increase her dosage. Since taking [n.n], she has had a noticeable decrease in blood sugar every morning when she tests it.

—L131, Indianapolis, IN

DIGESTION, DIARRHEA, PANCREATITIS

Within a week of starting [n.n], I noticed a marked improvement. It cleaned my facial skin of bumps, healed my lacerated tongue, and cured my indigestion. It has calmed down my pancreas and stopped my diarrhea. I had been easily winded and chronically tired, and I find that [n.n] has increased my endurance.

—R79, Rock Hill, SC

STOMACH GAS

My sister was having stomach problems. She had X rays taken, and was told she had a lot of trapped gas. She tried everything, but nothing seemed to help. I gave her some [n.n], and within 10 minutes she began to get release from that trapped gas. [n.n] is truly a blessing.

—L70, Texas

HEARTBURN

For many years, I have suffered from stomach pain and heartburn due to a hyperacidic stomach and sluggish digestion. [n.n] has improved my acid stomach problem 100 percent! I no longer have to take any stomach medication. In only a few days, I was feeling better all over. This is all the more welcome, as I have a slow thyroid as well.

—R76, Indian Lake, NY

PLATELET COUNT

I have been battling leukemia for eight years. At one point my platelet count was down to 5,000, and the doctors wanted to take my spleen out. They found plenty of platelets in my bone marrow, but it seemed my spleen was destroying them. At that time, I was put on Prednisone. When I started [n.n], my platelet count was "up" to 35,000 (250,000 is normal.) Four days later, I went off my medication, relying completely on [n.n]. One month later, my count was the same as with the medication. The end of the second month, it had come up 155,000. Stay tuned!

—R73, Sonora, CA

PHYSICAL AND MENTAL HEALTH IMPROVED

Since I have been taking [n.n], I have noticed my mental and physical health improve in so many ways. Increased energy and stamina have helped me recover from a mild depression. I am more alert, have greater clarity of mind, and need less sleep. I have noticed an improved body odor, and various skin rashes have cleared up. In fact, my skin texture overall is much improved.

—R9, Ann Arbor, MI

PET'S SKIN RASH

Asa, a large hunting dog, usually enjoyed very good health. However, a skin rash had become progressively worse, as he used his teeth in an attempt to relieve the itching. His owner, a [n.n] user, had tried several medications, but all to no effect. When she began giving him a daily dose of [n.n], the rash disappeared within a week.

—L126

PRE-MENSTRUAL SYNDROME

Before I started taking [n.n], I had cramps, headaches, irritability, emotional ups and downs, allergy symptoms, digestive problems, and chronic constipation. [n.n] relieved my constipation within a short time, and soon after that I began to see an improvement in many of my other symptoms. I have been taking [n.n] for five months now, and I feel so much better in the two weeks before my period. I now have very light or mild cramps, no irrationality, and my emotions stay on an even keel, thanks to [n.n].

—R35, Chino, CA

MENOPAUSE, ARTHRITIS

I consulted my gynecologist about my menopausal symptoms two years ago. At that time I decided against the estrogen and progesterone therapy and decided to rely on vitamin E and other supplements. Since I started taking [n.n], I feel better over all, with more energy. I began to see results within about two weeks. Not only do I have fewer hot flashes, but my arthritis is better.

—Rid, Orange, CA

ULCER AND SHOULDER PAIN GONE

My goal in taking [n.n] was simple: I wanted to regain my health. My ulcer and pain in my shoulder are gone and I feel much more relaxed and level-headed. I need less sleep and have more energy than ever. I can honestly say I feel like I'm 18 again—according to the calendar, I'm 32! I thank God for [n.n].

—R225 Sherwood Park, Alberta

OSTEOPOROSIS AND MUSCLE SPASMS

I started taking [n.n] about 10 days ago, and almost immediately began to feel better. I have osteoporosis, and had severe muscle spasms, crackling bones, and aches and pains all over my body. Now I sleep like a log and have almost no muscle spasms. The aches and pains are definitely leaving. I am filled with wonder and praise as I experience this marvelous healing that is taking place in my body each day.

—L63, San Antonio, TX

HEADACHES, EYESIGHT, ENERGY LEVEL, APPEARANCE

I had a heart attack two years ago, and since then have suffered from weakness, tiredness, and a tendency to get a headache whenever I read for more than a few minutes. [n.n] has changed all that. Now I can work faster and for longer periods and am glad to prepare meals. My energy lasts longer, my outlook is good, and I even look younger — less wrinkles on my face. My eyes have greatly improved so that I can read and don't get a headache.

—L93, Phoenix, AZ

PARKINSON'S DISEASE

Since starting on [n.n], I have more energy and a sense of well-being. I have even noticed a slight decrease in the shaking of my legs from Parkinson's disease.

—R55, San Antonio, TX

WARTS

I have had a continuing problem with warts on my hand. I had them burned off at the doctor's office and they still came back. That is only one of many different things I have tried. After only six weeks of taking [n.n], my warts are gone! I can hardly believe it, after everything else I tried had failed.

—L228, Madison, WI

FAT AND TIRED

I've been taking [n.n] for seven months, a heaping teaspoon every day. If you could have seen me before, you just wouldn't believe the difference in energy. I was 41, fat, and always tired. I've lost weight, I definitely need less sleep, and I generally feel 100 percent better. Now I eat "live" foods, I take [n.n], and I just can't believe how great I feel. I try to tell everyone about [n.n].

—R72, Santa Monica, CA

CHAPTER XII

Feeling the Difference

HOW TO TAKE GREEN BARLEY

If, after reading this book and being convinced of the attributes of green barley juice, you are ready to try it, then you are about to experience a whole new realm of health and well-being as you join the many users who say, "I wouldn't be without it — I really feel the difference!"

WHAT NOT TO DO

Your green barley powder is bursting with "live" enzymes and co-enzymes (vitamins) that will be destroyed if you "heat" it or freeze it. Therefore:

- DO NOT expose it to sunlight, air, or heat.
- DO NOT mix it with anything hot.
- DO NOT refrigerate it.
- USE ONLY a DRY spoon for getting the powder from the jar.

FOR BEST RESULTS

- Green barley is taken 30 minutes before or two hours after a meal — always on an empty stomach
- Healthy adults can use daily: 1 to 2 teaspoon servings of green barley powder dissolved in 6 to 8 ounces of water, fruit juice, or milk.

• If you notice detoxification symptoms, it might be best to LOWER your usage for a few days, then go back to a one teaspoon serving and add more gradually.

• If you have a chronic health problem (especially a degenerative disease such as arthritis, cancer, diabetes, or a heart condition, etc.,) many people have reported feeling better by using two teaspoons *three times a day,* always observing the guidelines about taking it on an empty stomach.

• Very small children (one-year-old, for example) often are given 1/4 teaspoon daily, older children 1/2 teaspoon a day, and teenagers one teaspoon or (whatever an adult would take). During times of illness, these amounts may be safely and greatly increased for short periods of time, according to Dr. Hagiwara.

• For adults, 20 grams, or about 10 teaspoons daily is considered by Dr. Hagiwara to be the maximum safe number of servings. A number of people, however, have reported taking more than this for short periods with good results.

IT TAKES TIME

Some people find that taking green barley at bedtime causes them to be too energized to sleep well. Others find it a perfect "nightcap"— make sure you have some leeway for experimentation before trying it!

If you "feel bad" after starting to take your green barley drink, rejoice! This may very well indicate that your body is initiating the "dump and rebuild" cycle known as detoxification. If you do experience detoxification symptoms, *reduce your intake* for a day or two, but do not stop taking it.

Last but not least, allow at least 16 to 24 or more weeks to really feel the difference.* Green barley leaves are not magic; rather, they are an excellent cell food. Given adequate time, dramatic results are frequently reported when directions are carefully and faithfully followed.

*Don't be discouraged if it takes eight months to one year before you see the results you want to experience.

LIVE FOODS MAKE LIVE PEOPLE;
DEAD FOODS MAKE DEAD PEOPLE

Genesis 1:29 KJV "And God said, Behold, I have given you every herb bearing seed, which is upon the face of all the earth, and every tree, in the which is the fruit of a tree yielding seed; to you it shall be for meat." (This statement was made to Adam and Eve.) From this we see that the original diet that God planned for man is what we would call a vegetarian diet:

EAT:

• All beans/ legumes/ lentils/ seeds & nuts. (These are your main protein foods.)

• All whole grains. (Barley/ rice/ wheat/ oats/ millet/ corn/ spelt/ amaranth — any natural grain. Use only whole grain breads. Boxed cereals are not whole grain.)

• All fresh vegetables and fruits. (Eat as many of them raw as you can tolerate. Frozen or canned veggies and fruits are better than none!)

• Distilled or reverse osmosis water only. (6 to 8 glasses daily: this is very important.)

• The key to disease prevention and/or cure is to eat a wide variety of veggies and fruits and whole grains. The wider the better.

OMIT FROM YOUR DIET: *(It only takes about 8 months to one year to turn sick cells to healthy cells.)*

• All meat (ALL flesh, including fish and fowl, and especially pork. See note on back of page.)

• All milk products (Unless you can buy certified, unpasteurized milk.) See Proverbs 27:27.

• Eggs (Unless you can buy fertile farm eggs — then 3 to 5 per week maximum.)

• "Man-made" products of all kinds, ("Designer foods" — like Cool Whip — are dead foods. Dead foods make dead people.)

• Most canned goods. (Naturally a few won't kill you.)

• All white sugar and baked goods using white flour (Use whole wheat flour and honey, maple syrup, molasses, fruit juice concentrates, dates, and raisins, etc. to sweeten.)

• All soft drinks. (They contain phosphoric acid, too much sugar and artificial products which soften bones and cause many other health problems.)

• All fruit juices except freshly squeezed ones. (They have too much sugar for sick cells unless you dilute them about half with water.)

• Eat NO margarine. (It is "plastic-like" and plugs arteries. Butter is OK in small amounts.)

• Water from your tap. (Chlorine and heavy metals produce free-radicals which produce carcinogens.)

• High fat foods. (Fried foods, sandwich meats like bologna, mayonnaise, snack foods, nuts in large amounts, doughnuts, potato and other chips, etc.)

• Use cold pressed virgin olive oil or canola oil in cooking.

• Coffee. (Not more than 1-2 cups per day. None if you have cancer. Use hot water with a slice of lemon. This will help cleanse the liver, kidneys, and bladder.)

Of course, rest, exercise and a positive mental attitude are also very important components of a healthy lifestyle.

READ:

I Co. 6:19	Gen. 1:29	Deut. 6:10-13	Prov. 27:27
I Co. 10:31	Lev. 3:17	Judges 13:14	Lev. 7:23
Phil. 3:18-19	Prov. 25:27	Deut. 32:15	Prov. 21:17
Gen. 1:11	Prov. 29:29	Ps. 141:3-4	Prov. 3:3-4

ADDITIONAL RAW, ORGANICALLY GROWN, WHOLE, "LIVE" FOOD PRODUCTS THAT PROMOTE THE HEALTHY CELL CONCEPT:

- 2-6 teaspoons of BarleyGreen a day.* Take 30 minutes before a meal or 2 hours afterward in water or juice.
- 4 glasses a day of freshly squeezed vegetable and fruit combinations. (Use carrots as the basic ingredient - as a meal, with a meal, or in-between meals.)
- 2 packages or heaping teaspoons or more of Just Carrots. (If you do not make fresh juices.)
- 2 Superzymes (chewed) before each meal.
- 2 glasses of Willard Water. (Add 1 oz. of Willard Water to 1 gallon of distilled or reverse-osmosis water.)
- At least 2 heaping teaspoons of Herbal Fiberblend. (A dirty colon produces and sustains disease.) Be sure to drink lots of water.
- 1 teaspoon of Redibeets. (May be added to other food concentrates, i.e., Just Carrots and BarleyGreen.)

* If you consider yourself chronically ill, you may find 10 teaspoons of BarleyGreen a day helpful. Take 2 teaspoons every 2 hours 5 times a day, always on an empty stomach. (Start with 1 tsp. 30 min. before breakfast; then 2 tsp's — 1 before breakfast and 1 at 3 pm, later 3 tsp's etc.)

BIBLIOGRAPHY AND FOOTNOTES

CHAPTER 1
1. *Proceeding of the Connecticut Medical Society for 1850.* Bound pamphlets printed in Norwich & Hartford, Vol. 1244, p. 53.

2. Atkins, Robert C., M.D., *Dr. Atkins' Health Revolution,* Houghton Mifflin Company, Boston, Mass., 1988, p.26.

3. *The Impact of Nutrition On the Health of Americans,* The Bard College Center, Annandale-on-Hudson, New York, The Medicine & Nutrition Project, Report No.1, The Ford Foundation, July, 1981, p. II/23.

4. Atkins, op. cit., p. 59.

CHAPTER 2
1. *Statistical Abstract of the U.S., U.S. Department of Commerce Bureau of the Census,* 1995, Chart 225, p. 147.

2. *The Book of Health Secrets,* Boardman Classics, N.Y., N.Y. 1989, p. 147.

3. Dean Black, Ph D., *Health at the Crossroads,* Tapestry Press, Springville, Utah, p. 49.

4. Brent O. Hafen, *Nutrition, Food and Weight Control,* Allyn and Bacon, Inc., Boston, 1981, p. 125. 4. FDA Special Report, op. cit., p. 5.

CHAPTER 3

1. Yoshihide Hagiwara, M.D., *Green Barley Essence,* Keats Publishing Co., New Canaan, 1985, p. XXVII.

2. John D. Kirschmann and Lavon Dunne, *Nutrition Almanac,* McGraw-Hill Book Company, New York, 2nd Ed., 1984, p. 235.

3. Wesley Marx, "Seaweed, the Ocean's Unsung Gift," *Reader's Digest,* Vol. 124, No. 746, Jun. 1984, p. 48.

4. Peter Bradford and Montse Bradford, *Cooking With Sea Vegetables,* Thorson's Publishing Group, Wellingborough, 1985, p. 60.

5. Kirschmann and Dunne, op. cit., p. 251.

6. Joseph Kadans, *Encyclopedia of Fruits, Vegetables, Nuts, and Seeds for Healthful Living,* Parker Publishing Co., Inc. W. Nyack, 1973, p. 73.

7. Nelson Coons, *Using Plants in Healing,* Rodale Press, Emmaus, 1963, p. 227.

8. Dr. Bernard Jensen, *Foods that Heal,* Avery Publishing Group, Inc., Garden City Park, NY, 1988, p. 9.

CHAPTER 4

1. William P. Pinkston, Jr., *Biology,* Bob Jones University Press, Greenville, 1980, p. 73.

2. Ibid. p. 897.

3. Arthur Guyton, *Textbook of Medical Physiology,* W. B. Saunders Co., Philadelphia, pp. 896-898.

4. Guyton, op. cit., p. 12.

5. Hans Selye, M.D., *The Stress of Life,* McGraw-Hill, NY, 1978, pp. xi-xvii.

6. Guyton, op. cit., p. 370.

7. Lawrence Lauch, M.D., *Metabolics,* 1974, p. 9.

CHAPTER 5

1. National Institute of Health, "Understanding the Immune System," U.S. Dept. of Health and Human Services, NIH Publication 85-529, reprinted July 1985, p. 2.

2. Ibid, p. 4.

3. Bruce Harstead, "Immune Augmentation Therapy," *Journal of*

the International Academy of Preventive Medicine, Vol. 9, No. 1, Aug. 1985, p. 9.

4. Jaret, Peter, "Our Immune System: The Wars Within," *National Geographic Magazine,* Vol. 169, No. 6, June 1986, p. 706.

5. Weiner, Michael A., Ph.D., *Maximum Immunity,* Pocket Books, New York, 1986, pp. 21-22.

6. NIH, p. 4.

7. Agatha Thrash, M.D., Lecture Notes, Yucci Pines Institute, Seal, AL. 1983.

8. Weiner, p. 82.

9. Ibid, p. 85.

10. Ibid, p. 86.

11. Ibid, p. 86.

12. Ibid, pp. 108-109.

13. William Beisel, et al "Single-Nutrient Effects on Immunologic Function," Journal of American Medical Association, Vol. 245, No. 1, Jan. 2, 1981, p. 55.

14. Weiner, p. 111.

15. Ibid, p. 112.

16. *JAMA,* op. cit., p. 55.

17. Ibid.

18. Weiner, p. 114.

19. *JAMA,* op. cit., p. 55.

20. Weiner, p. 117.

21. Ibid, p. 121.

22. Ibid. p. 122.

23. Weiner, p. 127.

24. Ibid.

CHAPTER 6

1. Dr. J.A. Driskell, Professor and Head, Department of Human Nutrition and Foods Virginia Polytechnic Institute and State University.

2. Lois Mattox Miller, "Chlorophyll for Healing," *Science News Letter* March 15, 1941, p. 170.

3. Ibid, p. 170.

4. G.A. Hendry and O.T. Jones, "Haems and Chlorophylls: Comparisons of Function and Formation," *Journal of Medical Genetics,* 1980, Fe. 17 (1) p. 14.

5. Benjamin Gruskin, "Chlorophyll—Its Therapeutic Place in Acute and Suppurative Diseases," *American Journal of Surgery,* July 1940, p. 50.

6. Paul Sack and Robert Barnard, "Studies on Hemagglutinating and Inflammatory Properties of Exudate from Nonhealing Wounds & Their Inhibition by Chlorophyll Derivatives," *New York State Journal of Medicine,* Oct. 15, 1955, Vol. 55, p. 2952.

7. Ibid p. 2955.

8. Gruskin, p. 54.

9. Ibid, p. 54.

10. Leonard Engel, "Can Chlorophyll Stop 'B.O.'?" *Science Digest,* October 1952, Vol. 32, p. 39.

11. Lawrence W. Smith, "The Present Status of Topical Chlorophyll Therapy," *New York State Journal of Medicine,* July 15, Vol. 55, p. 20-44.

12. Richard Young & Joseph Beregi, "Use of Chlorophyllin in Care of Geriatric Patients," *American Geriatrics Society Journal,* Jan. 1980, Vol. 28, No. 1, p. 47.

13. Milap Nahatal et al, "Effect of Chlorophyllin on Urinary Odor in Incontinent Geriatric Patients," *Drug Intelligence & Clinical Pharmacy,* Oct. 1983, Vol. 17, p. 734.

14. R. Tawashi, et al, "Effect of Sodium Copper Chlorophyllin on the Formation of Calcium Oxalate Crystals in Rat Kidney," *Investigative Urology,* Sept. 1980, Vol. 18, No. 2, p. 90.

CHAPTER 7

1. Arthur C. Guyton, M.D. *Textbook of Medical Physiology,* W.B. Saunders Co., Philadelphia, 1981, pp. 448-450.

2. Rubard Leek, PH.D., "Acidosis and Alkalosis: Symptoms and Treatments," *The Nutrition and Dietary Consultant,* Oct. 1985.

3. Margaret Justin, et all, *Foods,* Houghton Mifflin Co., Boston, 4th Ed., pp. 42-43.

4. Ibid, p. 26.

5. Margaret Chaney and Margaret Ross, *Nutrition,* Houghton Mifflin Co., Boston, 7th Ed., p. 326.

6. Agatha Thrash, M.D., *Eat for Strength — Not For Drunkenness,* Yucci Pines Institute, Seale, AL. p. 182.

7. Leek, op. cit., p. 14.

8. Robert H. Garrison, Jr., *The Nutrition Desk Reference,* Keats Publishing Co., New Canaan, 1985, p. 106.

9. Ibid.

10. Ibid.

11. Ibid.

12. Ibid.

13. Leek, op. cit., p. 15.

CHAPTER 8

1. Howell, Edward, *The Status of Food Enzymes in Digestion and Metabolism,* (Chicago: National Enzyme Co., 1946) p. 72

2. Howell, op. cit., p. Xl.

3. Ibid, p. 29.

4. Ibid, p. 107

5. Howell, Edward, *Enzyme Nutrition,* Avery Publishing Group, Inc., Wayne, NJ, 1985.

6. Ibid, p. 109

7. Ibid, p. 112.

8. Ibid, p. 43.

9. Ibid, p. 50.

10. William Campbell Douglas, M.D., *The Milk of Human Kindness,* Last Laugh Publishers, Marietta, Ga., 1985, p. 42-43.

CHAPTER 9

1. Yoshihide Hagiwara, M.D., "Prevention of Aging and Adult Diseases and Methods of Longevity and Good Health," an abstract, lecture given at Pacific Beach Hotel, Honolulu, April 13, 1984, p. 5.

2. Kazuhiko Kubota, Ph.D., "Scientific Investigations on Young Barley Juice Powder," Lecture given at Pacific Beach Hotel, Honolulu, April 13, 1984, p. 1.

3. Hagiwara, lecture, op. cit., p. 6.

4. Yasuo Hotta, DS., "Stimulation of DNA Repair Synthesis by P_4D_1, One of the Novel Components of Barley Extracts," lecture, Pacific Beach Hotel, Honolulu 4/13/84.

5. Ibid.

6. Ibid.

7. Ibid.

8. Irwin Fridovich, "The Biology of Superoxide and of Superoxide Dismutases—in Brief," *Progress in Clinical and Biological Research,* Vol. 51, 1981, p. 159.

9. Thomas Kensler, et.al., "Inhibition of Tumor Promotion by a Biomimetic Superoxide Dismutase," *Science,* Vol. 231, Jul. 1, 1983, pp. 75-77.

CHAPTER 10

1. Adrianne Bendich, Carotenoids and the Immune Response, *Journal of Nutrition,* 119: 112-115, 1989.

2. Ibid.

3. *Science News,* Vol. 135, June 3, 1989, pg. 348.

4. Hagiwara, op cit., p. 80.

5. Ibid., p. 58.

POSTSCRIPT

Years of study and experience have fully confirmed that Nature has provided a wide variety of delicious and nutritious foods perfectly designed for the growth maintenance and repair of all tissue. This truth was magnified exponentially to me as I recently read and understood results of years of research by a number of Botanists from various countries of the world.

Beginning in the later part of the 19th century, and continuing until today, scientific investigations by the hundreds, in different fields, have shown us undeniably that everything in the universe radiates electromagnetic waves which can be identified as sound, color, form, movement, perfume, temperature and "innate awareness."

While all plant radiations differ from one another (like our thumb prints and snow flakes!) they have a time when the radiations are at their peak. In most cases this coincides with the height of their maturity, which is also near a full moon.

Now buckle your seatbelts and trust me. What I want to share is purely scientific evidence but it validates perfectly the account in Genesis 1:29. God told Adam and Eve, "Behold I have given you every plant yielding seed that is on the surface of all the earth and every tree which has fruit yielding seed; for you this is meat."

A botanist from France developed an instrument called a biometer which enabled him to measure frequencies being emitted from foods, in centimeters and angstroms.*

The wavelengths coming from the foods could tell both their freshness and the vitality or strength of the food.

Now for the part that is thrilling to me. Without exception, the foods with the highest number of angstroms are the foods God told Adam and Eve to eat. Here is the list:

10,000 to 8,500 angstroms — Barley, wheat, oats and other grains; butter and garlic; fruits and vegetables if eaten fresh; olive oil; and legumes, lentils and beans.

---

* *An angstrom is 100 millionth of a centimeter - a unit in measuring the length of light waves.*

6,500 down to 3,000 angstroms — fresh milk, wine, peanut oil, boiled fruits and vegetables, unrefined cane sugar, canned fish and dried foods.

No angstrom foods — coffee, tea, chocolate, jams, cheeses, white bread, day-old milk, margarines, jellies, canned fruits, canned vegetables, alcohols, liquors, white sugar, bleached white four, pasteurized fruit and vegetable juices.

Space does not permit more about food angstroms in this edition. But please, accept the facts whether or not you fully understand the science behind them.

We were designed to thrive on raw fruits, vegetables, grains, nuts, seeds, berries, and the beans, legumes and lentils. These are the foods that energize our bodies, build strong immune systems, heal us when we are sick and make us radiantly healthy.

Gamble on it! What do you have to lose?

Another fact about angstroms in food is worth sharing. Dr. Marcus McCausland of London reported to the World Congress of Science and Religion in Rome (1979) the following information. He measured the angstroms being emitted from a loaf of freshly baked bread. The bread was then blessed by saying a prayer over it. Upon remeasuring the bread, it was found that the number of angstroms being emitted had increased above the original reading.

There is both Old and New Testament precedent for saying "grace" before meals. In Samuel 9:13 we are told that the people were not allowed to eat until the prophet came to bless the food. In the New Testament there are four references to saying grace over a meal. (See Mt. 14:19; 15:36; Acts 27:35; and I Cor. 11:24.)

The two Scriptures in Matthew record two different incidents in which Jesus commanded large crowds to sit down on the grass. Then looking up to heaven, Jesus blessed a small number of loaves of bread and fish, broke them and fed multitudes of people (thousands), with full baskets left over.

Another of my favorite Scriptures is Ex. 23:25. "And ye shall serve the Lord your God, and He shall bless thy bread and thy water; and I will take sickness away from the midst of thee."

I close with this challenge. Serve God with all of your heart; He is a God who keeps His promises.

INDEX

BOOKS BY DR. MARY RUTH SWOPE

Green Leaves of Barley: Nature's Miracle Rejuvenator - Updated Edition *New '96*	$9.95
Surviving the 20th Century Diet: Scientific Solutions To A Diet Gone Wrong	
New for '96 - The Abridged Version of Green Leaves of Barley	$6.95
Some Gold Nuggets in Nutrition - *Newly Updated for '96*	$4.00
Green Leaves of Barley: French Translation	$9.95
Green Leaves of Barley: Spanish or Chinese Translation	$6.95
The Spiritual Roots of Barley	$5.00
Are You Sick & Tired of Feeling Sick & Tired?	$5.00
Listening Prayer	$5.00
Listening Prayer: Spanish or Chinese Translation	$6.95
Fasting...Physical and Spiritual Benefits	$1.00
Bless Your Children Everyday	$9.95
Bless Your Children Everyday: Spanish, Chinese or Russian Translation	$6.95

OTHER RECOMMENDED BOOKS

Green Barley Essence by Dr. Yoshihide Hagiwara	$10.95
Green Barley Essence - Abridged Version	$3.95
God's Way To Ultimate Health by Reverend George H. Malkmus	$17.95
Why Christians Get Sick by Reverend George H. Malkmus	$8.95
Country Life Vegetarian Cookbook edited by Diana J. Fleming	$9.95
Antioxidants, Coenzyme Q10, Ginko Biloba by Dr. E.S. Wagner, Ph.D.	$1.00
Wagner Book "Trio" - (1 each of the above)	$2.95
Of These Ye May Eat Freely by JoAnn Rachor	$3.95
Fit As A Fiddle by Jeani McKeever	$6.95
The Coming Revival by Dr. Bill Bright	$11.95
Aqua Vitae - (The Story of Dr. John W. Willard: Catalyst Altered Water) by Roy M. Jacobsen	$10.95
Cleansing the Body and the Colon by Teresa Schumacher & Toni Schumacher Lund	$3.95
The New Superantioxidant - Plus by Richard A. Passwater, Ph.D.	$3.95

VIDEO TAPES

Nutrition Update...BarleyGreen by Swope/Darbro	(30 minutes)	$15.00
What to Eat & What Not To Eat by Dr. Swope	(60 minutes)	$20.00
It's Not Too Late: Nutritional Update by Swope/McKeever	(58 minutes)	$20.00
Using Nutrition as Medicine by Swope/McKeever	(43 minutes)	$20.00
Cancer Doesn't Scare Me Anymore by Lorraine Day, M.D.	(77 minutes)	$20.00

INTERNATIONAL ORDERS - U.S. FUNDS ONLY
All Prices Subject to Change Without Prior Notice

SHIPPING AND HANDLING

$ AMOUNT	U.S.	CAN	INT'L		$ Amount	U.S.	CAN	INT'L
$0 and up	$3	$6	Call	Other Case Prices By Request	$75 and up	$9	$18	Call
$10 and up	$4	$8	Us		$100	$11	Call	Us
$20 and up	$5	$10	Call		Over $100		Us	
$30 and up	$6	$12	Us		Repeat Chgs			
$40 and up	$7	$14	Call		Case GLB	$15	Call	Call
$50 and up	$8	$16	Us		Case BYC	$15	Us	Us

NAME _____ AMOUNT ENCLOSED
ADDRESS_____ _____
CITY/STATE/ZIP _____
PHONE (_____)_____ *PLEASE CALL US WITH ANY QUESTIONS*